THIS MAY HURT A BIT

Stephen Skyvington

Foreword by Dr. Brian Day

THIS MAY HURT A BIT

Reinventing Canada's Health Care System

DUNDURN
TORONTO

Cover image: istock.com/malerapaso
Printer: Webcom, a division of Marquis Book Printing Inc.

Library and Archives Canada Cataloguing in Publication

Skyvington, Stephen, author
     This may hurt a bit : reinventing Canada's health care
system / Stephen Skyvington ; foreword by Dr. Brian Day.

Includes bibliographical references and index.
Issued also in print and electronic formats.
ISBN 978-1-4597-4243-7 (softcover).--ISBN 978-1-4597-4244-4
(PDF).--ISBN 978-1-4597-4245-1 (EPUB)

     1. Medical care--Canada. 2. Medical policy--Canada.
3. Public health--Canada. 4. National health insurance--Canada.
5. Health care reform--Canada. I. Day, Brian, 1947-, writer of
foreword II. Title.

RA395.C3S58 2019   362.10971   C2018-906145-6
                                             C2018-906146-4

1 2 3 4 5   23 22 21 20 19

 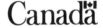 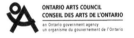

We acknowledge the support of the **Canada Council for the Arts**, which last year invested $153 million to bring the arts to Canadians throughout the country, and the **Ontario Arts Council** for our publishing program. We also acknowledge the financial support of the **Government of Ontario**, through the **Ontario Book Publishing Tax Credit** and **Ontario Creates**, and the **Government of Canada**.

Nous remercions le **Conseil des arts du Canada** de son soutien. L'an dernier, le Conseil a investi 153 millions de dollars pour mettre de l'art dans la vie des Canadiennes et des Canadiens de tout le pays.

Care has been taken to trace the ownership of copyright material used in this book. The author and the publisher welcome any information enabling them to rectify any references or credits in subsequent editions.

— *J. Kirk Howard, President*

The publisher is not responsible for websites or their content unless they are owned by the publisher.

Printed and bound in Canada.

VISIT US AT

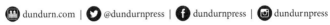

dundurn.com | @dundurnpress | dundurnpress | dundurnpress

Dundurn
3 Church Street, Suite 500
Toronto, Ontario, Canada
M5E 1M2

To my friends and family

Status quo, you know, is Latin for the "mess we're in."
— *Ronald Reagan*

The difference between a politician and a statesman is that a politician thinks about the next election while the statesman thinks about the next generation.
— *James Freeman Clarke*

Innovation distinguishes between a leader and a follower.
— *Steve Jobs*

Politics is the art of looking for trouble, finding it everywhere, diagnosing it incorrectly, and applying the wrong remedies.
— *Groucho Marx*

CONTENTS

$(\!\!\!=\!\!\!\!\!\blacksquare\!\!\!\!\!=\!\!\!-$ FOREWORD $-\!\!\!\blacksquare\!\!\!\!\!\blacksquare\!\!\!\!)$

In Canada, perhaps more than in any other country, politics exerts an over-powering and negative influence when it comes to discussing and debating health care policy. It is fitting, therefore, that an experienced political guru, Stephen Skyvington, has written this concise but challenging and insightful book on his vision for improving a health scheme that is no longer fulfilling its promises.

Stephen has a long history of involvement with health care policy and politics. He describes how, in Canada, political diversions and considerations have negatively impacted all attempts at meaningful reform and improve-ment. Canada has suffered from this politicization. This book approaches potential solutions in a rational and organized way.

The author also has many years of experience as both an insider and outsider in the bureaucracies that govern medical politics and health policy in Canada. He has extensive professional involvement with doctors and their medical organizations. Although not a physician, in this book he has adopted an approach that we doctors use in the diagnosis and treatment of a sick patient: he has compiled a detailed history of the problem, followed by a comprehensive examination and investigation, and finished with a prescription for the treatment of the many ills that exist in Canadian health care.

In this book he describes how the current "system" evolved, pointing out that there really is no such thing as a "Canadian health system." Each province and territory has its own health ministry and bureaucracy. The potential for these to have served as models, where different innovations could have been evaluated to provide lessons that other provinces could learn from, has not been realized. Instead, the many different schemes have had their potential for improvement stifled by the Canada Health Act. New initiatives have focused on those that benefit governments and their bureaucracies, rather than patients.

Also discussed is the role of the federal government in impeding provincial governments' attempts to initiate necessary reforms. Health costs are currently rising at a much greater rate than the economy can sustain. B.C. has enacted the five principles of the Canada Health Act into provincial legislation and has added "sustainability" as a sixth principle. An undocumented principle is the widely applied principle of enforced rationing.

Stephen makes a good suggestion that "quality" should be added as a sixth principle to the Canada Health Act. Unfortunately, governments currently enforce public administration and blatantly ignore the other principles (comprehensiveness, universality, portability, and accessibility). Their record suggests they would ignore the principle of quality.

An informative chapter deals with the hypocrisy of those who, at the expense of patients, support the status quo. Hypocrisy is perhaps one of the worst vices of all, especially when practised by those in authority. The activities of certain organized groups and ideologues, including some physicians who achieve positions of power, are disturbing.

Canadian governments are unremorseful as they trample on the rights of patients. In the 2011 safe injection site case, the Supreme Court of Canada stated, "Where a law creates a risk to health by preventing access to health care, a deprivation of the right to security of the person is made out.... Where the law creates a risk not just to the health but also to the lives of the claimants, the deprivation is even clearer." Canadians are subjected to a "health system" that the same court stated is causing the suffering and deaths of Canadians. It is a court that struck down laws that made abortion, same-sex marriage, safe injection sites, and medically assisted dying unlawful.

It also gave prisoners the right to vote. These are not the rulings of some right-wing legal entity.

This book analyzes government policies that deal with matters of life and death, pointing out that Canada is alone in enforcing legal control over its citizens' bodies. The late Stanley Hartt QC, who was a lawyer for the Senate intervenors in the 2005 Chaoulli case, opined that the only legal defence that could justify the status quo would be that wait-lists for access to care had been eliminated in Canada.

Canada's health system is failing its most vulnerable citizens and our governments have avoided all responsibility for their failings. Their strategy has been to create tax-funded health commissions that have squandered hundreds of millions of dollars without any results. The solutions are seen in best practices of the many countries that deliver universal care far more effectively and efficiently than we do in Canada. Governments have, with the support of special interest groups, abrogated their duty to care for patients.

A few years ago, Dennis Leung of the *Ottawa Citizen* wrote, "It is fundamentally perverse for government to effectively ban us from contributing directly to most types of health care, on the basis that the care must be provided by government, then fail to deliver the care." That "perverse" situation is faced by millions of Canadians today. The concept that the state should own and control your bodily integrity is unique to Canada.

Stephen Skyvington has described the outcome when governments assume monopoly control of the funding and delivery of hospital and physician services. He has outlined practical and effective measures to address governments' failed promises to patients. This book deserves your attention — your future health may depend on it.

— Dr. Brian Day, M.R.C.P., F.R.C.S.,
orthopedic surgeon, health researcher, and past president
of the Canadian Medical Association
December 2018

⊶— PROLOGUE —⊷

THE ROOTS OF COINCIDENCE

They say every journey starts with but a single step. Our journey begins on December 12, 1983; that's when Canada's minister of health at the time, Monique Bégin, rose in the House of Commons to introduce the Canada Health Act. This particular piece of legislation, which would, among other things, ban "extra-billing" and eliminate user fees, was passed unanimously by Parliament in 1984, receiving royal assent on April 1.

A bad April Fool's joke, if ever there was one.

Politicians have used the Canada Health Act ever since it became law as a way of defining who we are as Canadians, frequently wrapping themselves in the flag and accusing those who are in favour of innovative new ways to fund medicare of being unpatriotic. Interest groups, particularly unions, have used perceived threats against the act as a way of raising money to fight critics, like Dr. Brian Day of British Columbia, who bravely brought a Charter challenge against the B.C. government in 2009 for failing to provide care in a timely manner. While Minister Bégin may have had the best of intentions, the fact remains that by giving birth to the Canada Health Act she opened up a Pandora's box of half-truths, misconceptions, and out-and-out lies that continue to impact the health care debate in this country three decades later.

Inspired by Monique Bégin's introduction of the Canada Health Act, Ontario's premier, and the leader of the Liberal Party, David Peterson, decided to go her one better by bringing forth the Health Care Accessibility Act in 1985. The bill, which was introduced on December 20, laid out the government's plan for implementing a ban on extra-billing. Ontario's doctors, through their representative, the Ontario Medical Association (OMA), argued that extra-billing should be left alone as it acted as a kind of safety valve, taking pressure off an already overburdened system. The premier and his attorney general, Ian Scott, rightly guessed that although the public generally loved their own doctors, they'd be willing to support the government so long as it positioned itself as the guardian and defender of medicare. The doctors fought back, organizing a series of job actions in the spring of 1986, but things fell apart when individual doctors and the Medical Reform Group started speaking out and distancing themselves from the OMA. Twenty-five days after it commenced, the strike ended and the modern era of doctor-bashing began in earnest. Clawbacks, unilateral fee cuts, and attempts by health ministers of all three parties to deliberately mislead the public about doctors' compensation would ultimately demoralize the medical profession. In one very public case, the government's actions led to the heartbreaking suicide of Dr. Tony Hsu, a pediatrician practising in Welland, Ontario, who took his life after an especially cruel and callous audit by the College of Physicians and Surgeons of Ontario's (CPSO) Medical Review Committee.

Nine years after the Ontario doctors' strike fizzled out, on March 29, 1995, to be precise, I was hired, much to my surprise, by the Ontario Medical Association. I say "much to my surprise," because the OMA kept postponing the interview. First, they wanted to meet with me, then they didn't. Then they did. In retrospect, this should have been a clue to what I was in for. But, at the time, I was desperate for a job, any job, and was willing to overlook just about anything in exchange for a regular paycheque.

A few days after I started, I arrived at my office to discover a modern-day "Night of the Long Knives" was under way. Twenty employees were either fired or quit, all on the same day, including my new boss and three-quarters of the public affairs and communications department, of which I was the newest member. Apparently, there'd been a staff revolt against the new chief executive officer, David Pattenden, who'd been hired the previous autumn.

The board backed the CEO, which meant those disgruntled staff members would be given the choice of either walking the plank on their own or being shown the door. While most everyone else around me was freaking out, I stayed calm as I saw an opportunity there. I spoke with David, who was keen on finding anyone who was willing to be his ally, and told him I could be his government relations guy while he was figuring out how to rebuild the public affairs and communications department. Thus began six and a half of the most interesting years of my life, as I, for all intents and purposes, became the doctors' lobbyist, a role I played until I left the OMA in the autumn of 2001 to form my own company.

•••

Three seemingly random and unrelated events: Monique Bégin introduces the Canada Health Act, David Peterson takes on Ontario's doctors, and I go to work for the Ontario Medical Association. Three events — two of which shaped Canada's health care system and political landscape, and a third that changed my life and the path I was on, as well as the way I would come to view things. No longer would I see doctors as a bunch of "fat cats," taking Wednesdays off to play golf, and driving around in big cars. No longer would I blindly put my faith in those running our country, assuming the ones in charge would always do what was best for us. No longer would I buy into the myth that Canada has the best health care system in the world.

Without these three events unfolding precisely the way they did, this book would not exist.

What This Book Is … (and Isn't)

Someone once said, "The person who consumes a meal is just as qualified to judge it as the person who prepared the meal." While it's true I never graduated from university — I attended York University from 1977 to 1980, studying fine arts and education, before leaving without a degree after three and a half years — and have never been a policy wonk or a member of a prestigious think tank, the fact remains I've been a patient, a caregiver, a lobbyist, and a player in the ever-evolving world of health care politics. So, when I say I know a thing or two about health care, especially when it comes to diagnosing what's wrong with Canada's health care system, you should trust me.

On a more personal level, I've witnessed first-hand the challenges and frustrations patients face when they find themselves in need of care. My brother Jim died of cancer — metastatic melanoma — in 1999, just a few days shy of his fiftieth birthday. My father died four years later, in 2003, of prostate cancer, having almost "stroked out" a couple of years earlier because of blood clots on the brain. My mother died in 2013, mostly of complications from pneumonia and sepsis, after having been misdiagnosed by the doctor on call at her local hospital as suffering from a bladder infection. She was eighty-four years old and in the early stages of dementia, having just been diagnosed six months previously. In her case, it's quite possible our health care system did mom a favour by hastening her end before things turned bad.

Still …

In 2015 it was my turn. The day began innocently enough. I'd walked the dogs, had a shower, and was just about to send a last few emails before leaving for a meeting with a potential client. All of a sudden, my heart started beating wildly. Now, this wasn't the first time this had happened. Back in 2012 I'd undergone a procedure to get what turned out to be a fairly serious case of atrial fibrillation under control. The operation was deemed a success and I was able to go on with my life pretty much as before. But what I was experiencing this morning was different. It was a V-tach attack, as it turned out — "ventricular tachycardia" is the exact term the doctors used, after zapping my heart back into something resembling a more normal rhythm. It was while riding in the back of the ambulance I decided I had to write this book before it was too late.

•••

Canada's health care system is complicated, no doubt about it. It's a minefield, full of people and groups with self-serving agendas and old-fashioned, out-of-date ideas that just don't work anymore. Many have come forward and offered their solutions. Regrettably, most of what they're proposing is impractical and not worth considering, to put it kindly. What's needed, in my view, is a plan that defines the problem in simple terms and offers *viable* solutions that will actually work in the real world. A plan whose foundation isn't based on what I like to call "magical thinking" — the sort of stuff being brought forward by the defenders of the status quo and deniers of the truth. By posing three simple questions — "How might we?"; "Why would we want to?"; and "What's stopping us from doing so?" — I show there is another way, a better way, to deliver and fund health care here in our country.

This May Hurt A Bit: Reinventing Canada's Health Care System is a book about big ideas. It's a book about "thinking outside the box" and not being afraid to try new things, things that, for the most part, have never been tried before here in Canada. Or, in some cases, haven't been tried for a very long time. It's a book that's meant to act as a blueprint of sorts, a plan that if implemented in whole — no cherry-picking, please — would provide a solid foundation on which to rebuild our failing health care system.

My motivation for writing this book is simple. I've been fortunate to have had a front-row seat during the past twenty-five years or so as politician after politician, and political party after political party, have tried to fix medicare here in Canada. For those of you who're hockey fans — and what true Canadian isn't? — it's been a little bit like watching those in charge try, and fail, to fix what's wrong with the Toronto Maple Leafs. But in the same way team president Brendan Shanahan and his management team have proven it *is* possible to do the impossible, by tearing down the team and rebuilding it from the bottom up, I believe we can blow up Canada's health care system and reinvent it so that we end up with something new and better.

Finally, and perhaps most importantly, I hope to take some of the emotion out of the debate. Now, no one loves this country more than I do. Unfortunately, my detractors would have you believe I have a hidden agenda, that my goal is to foist on Canada a U.S.-style, two-tier health care system. The irony, however, is that if we continue to keep our heads buried in the sand like we have for the past fifty years, trying to prop up a system that simply isn't sustainable, then we'll indeed end up with exactly what our neighbours to the south have: a health care system that's a bloody mess.

And none of us wants that.

(·——— PART I ———·)

BACK TO THE FUTURE

Canada, as a country, has always been somewhat star-struck. Maybe it's because Canadians are, as a whole, so gosh-darned polite and humble. Or maybe it's because we have such a massive inferiority complex we only feel validated if someone bigger and more important than us, say, someone with a huge international profile like U.S. senator and former presidential candidate Bernie Sanders, decides they need to start paying attention to what we're doing.

In the case of Senator Sanders, he made a much-ballyhooed trip to Canada in late October of 2017 at the invitation of Dr. Danielle Martin, vice-president of medical affairs and health system solutions at Women's College Hospital in Toronto, and Kathleen Wynne, premier of Ontario. Dr. Martin, who became a YouTube sensation in 2014 by taking on a Republican senator during a widely publicized appearance before a partisan U.S. Senate committee looking into the Patient Protection and Affordable Care Act (a.k.a. Obamacare), had recently published a book, entitled *Better Now: Six Big Ideas to Improve Health Care for All Canadians*, in which she suggested there was nothing seriously wrong with Canada's health care system that a Liberal dose of socialism (i.e., boatloads of money taken from the pockets of unsuspecting taxpayers) couldn't fix. Not surprisingly, the good senator, himself a dyed-in-the-wool socialist, was quick to latch onto Dr. Martin's nonsense.

Like something out of *Mr. Smith Goes to Washington*, or perhaps a strange and baffling episode of *The Twilight Zone*, we were treated to scene after scene of Senator Sanders being taken from one health care centre to the next — events all carefully orchestrated so that the beaming senator could witness one miracle after another. I couldn't help thinking how terribly appropriate it was that this truly naive and easily led visitor from the south had chosen to make his pilgrimage to Canada so close to Halloween. It was as if Dr. Martin and Premier Wynne were taking young Bernie door to door, smiling like Cheshire cats as he received treat after treat, which the little boy squirrelled away in his satchel so he could take each piece of candy out and savour it once he got back home.

Watching all this unfold, hour after hour, day after day, thanks in part to our ever-accommodating media, who apparently are incapable of asking probing, tough questions, I began to feel sorry for Sanders. Here was a man who'd built a reputation as something of a straight shooter, that rare breed of politician who actually cared about the truth, one who said what he meant and meant what he said. Sadly for Senator Sanders, he was being showered with "treats" by two used-car salespersons, who appeared to have no qualms about "tricking" the senator into believing that Canada has one of the best, if not *the* best, health care systems in the world. Never mind the shortages of doctors, nurses, and pharmacists. Never mind that many of our emergency departments are now operating well above 100 percent of their capacity, which has resulted in patients being stacked up on gurneys like so many planes on a runway, waiting for takeoff. And for God's sake, whatever you do, don't you dare mention wait times. After all, being a child of the 1960s, Bernie is not a young man anymore. We don't want to give him a heart attack.

If I'd been asked to meet with Senator Sanders, here's what I would have told him: "In order to know where you're going, you have to know where you've been."

Now, lots of people *think* they know how Canada's health care system came into being. "Tommy Douglas, the former premier of Saskatchewan and one-time leader of the New Democratic Party," they'll tell you, "was the father of Canadian medicare." They're wrong, but that's what pretty much everyone in this country has grown up believing. So much so that in a poll conducted by the Canadian Broadcasting Corporation in 2004, Douglas was named the "Greatest Canadian." Even more believe that they, and they alone, know what's in the Canada Health Act. They'll swear up and down, for instance, that one of the five principles of the act says medicare must be publicly funded. In fact, it says that medicare must be publicly *administered*. There's a big difference. This has resulted in Canada's health care landscape being littered with so much unhelpful rhetoric it's a wonder anyone can see the forest for the trees.

To help cut through some of this clutter, I thought it might be a good idea to look back at how we came to find ourselves in the mess we're in when it comes to health care. To this end, I'm going to focus on five things I believe were seminal in the building of our health care house of cards here in Canada, where it's become only too easy to fool ourselves into believing we do indeed have the best system in the world, even though the truth is far from that: Tommy Douglas and the Saskatchewan experiment; the Hall Commission and the introduction of medicare; the Canada Health Act; the Savings and Restructuring Act; and the Commitment to the Future of Medicare Act.

Starting with Tommy Douglas and the Saskatchewan experiment is something of a "no-brainer," of course, even if Douglas really wasn't medicare's father. After all, without this bold early attempt, it's entirely possible the rest of Canada's provinces might never have been convinced to dip their collective toes into the healing waters of medicare. Likewise, a closer examination of the mid-1960s commission overseen by Justice Emmett Hall is in order, if for no other reason than to show there were just as many Canadians against the creation of a national health care system as there were in favour. Which brings us to the Canada Health Act. While many feel the Canada Health Act has been something of an albatross around our necks, the very thing that's been stifling innovation and creativity and ultimately pulling us down these past thirty-plus years, the fact remains that its introduction was, without a doubt, one of the most important moments in our country's history. Finally, I'll take a look at two pieces of legislation that had big impacts here in Ontario when they were introduced and are still affecting our health care system today, as other provinces (Alberta, Quebec, and British Columbia, in particular) have gone on to bring forward their own versions of the bills. The Savings and Restructuring Act was brought in by the Mike Harris Conservatives in 1996, as part of their Common Sense Revolution. The Commitment to the Future of Medicare Act was the work of George Smitherman, Premier Dalton McGuinty's first health minister, after the Liberals defeated the Progressive Conservatives in 2003. In some ways, both of these pieces of legislation have had an even bigger impact on the health care environment in Ontario, and, indeed, in the rest of Canada, than even the Canada Health Act.

Tommy Douglas and the Saskatchewan Experiment

By now, just about everyone in Canada knows the story. When he was a young boy, Tommy Douglas fell and hurt his leg. Faced with amputation, as a result of his family not being able to afford the operation that would save his leg, the future premier of Saskatchewan was spared having to wear a prosthetic limb for the rest of his life when a renowned surgeon, Dr. R.J. Smith, offered to operate for free, so long as his medical students could watch. While grateful for Dr. Smith's timely intervention, Douglas made it clear years later that as far as he was concerned no child should ever have to depend upon the ability of his or her parents to raise the necessary funds to engage the services of a first-class surgeon, saying that had he been a rich man's son, he'd have had no problems getting the treatment he needed in a timely manner instead of having to depend upon chance for a cure.

Thus, the seed of medicare was planted.

Thomas "Tommy" Clement Douglas was born in Falkirk, Scotland. He immigrated to Canada with his family for a second time in 1918, having originally come over in 1910 before returning to Glasgow, Scotland, for a brief period following the outbreak of the First World War. An amateur boxer, a Baptist minister, and a politician, it seemed there was nothing the scrappy Douglas couldn't do, no challenge he wasn't willing to take on.

After being elected the first Co-operative Commonwealth Federation (CCF) premier of Saskatchewan in 1944, winning forty-seven of fifty-three seats, and forming the very first democratically elected socialist government in North America, Tommy Douglas rolled up his sleeves and got to work. During that first term, the new government created Saskatchewan's first publicly owned power company, which enabled the province to begin extending electrical services to remote farms and small towns and villages. The Douglas government also introduced Canada's first publicly owned auto insurance plan, as well as a program that offered free hospital care to all residents of the province — a first in North America. Before his inaugural term in office was over, Premier Douglas proudly ushered in the Saskatchewan Bill of Rights, and introduced legislation allowing the public service to unionize. Remarkably, the CCF would win four more majorities in Saskatchewan, making for a total of five in all. It was at last swept out of office in 1964, after Douglas had stepped down as premier in 1961 to become leader of the federal New Democratic Party.

Before leaving Saskatchewan for Ottawa, however, Tommy Douglas had one more trick up his sleeve — the introduction of universal health care coverage in Saskatchewan. Thanks to a booming economy and prudent fiscal stewardship, the Douglas government had managed to pay off the large public debt that had been left them by the previous Liberal government, resulting in a modest surplus for the province. This, coupled with a promise from the Diefenbaker government in Ottawa to give more money for medical care — fifty cents on the dollar — to any province that introduced a hospital plan, opened the door for the introduction of medicare in Saskatchewan.

The Saskatchewan Medical Care Insurance Act received royal assent in November of 1961, but implementation was delayed until July 1, 1962, by Douglas's successor, Woodrow Lloyd, to allow for a cooling-off period in the long and very public quarrel with the province's doctors, who were vehemently opposed to the plan. In spite of this delay, 90 percent of Saskatchewan's doctors went on strike on July 1, shutting down the health care system in the province for the next twenty-three days. The doctors had a number of concerns. Chief among them was a fear the medical profession would suffer significant losses of both income and autonomy. They were particularly worried that the government would interfere with the way doctors practised medicine, coming between them and their patients, or might even deny patients the right to choose their own doctor. Eventually, a truce was reached and the strike came to an end, thus ending the dispute — though the tension between doctors and their political masters would continue to percolate just below the surface for many years.

Ironically, it was this resistance by organized medicine that ensured the success of medicare in Saskatchewan, and ultimately paved the way for a similar program to be rolled out by the federal government all across Canada over the next decade. I believe I can explain why this was so. As someone who has worked with doctors for many years now, I've come to understand how physicians think and why they're often their own worst enemies. The answer is quite simple, really. Doctors, as a result of their training, know a great deal about a very limited field. They, even general and family practitioners, are society's ultimate specialists. Unfortunately, doctors tend to think they know a great deal about *everything*. They're convinced they are great negotiators. Or gifted public relations gurus. This is why when governments choose to act and make changes to something as complex and complicated as our health care system — as they are known to do every now and then — doctors will typically open their mouths in order to insert both feet without stopping to think about what they're saying and what the ramifications of their words might be.

This is precisely what happened in Saskatchewan in the early 1960s. One can't help but cringe at some of the tactics the medical profession used to try to make their case. They suggested, for instance, that the government would bring over the "garbage of Europe" to replace Canadian doctors. They burned Tommy Douglas in effigy and distributed pamphlets and posters portraying the CCF as a bunch of commies. Many shuttered their offices, and deliberately understaffed emergency departments, which may well have contributed to the tragic death of nine-month-old Carl Derhousoff on the first day of the strike. No wonder the public turned against doctors. Physicians made it easy for them to do so.

And yet, for a while there, it looked like the doctors were going to win the day with their anti-medicare campaign. Importing tactics first road-tested by the American Medical Association and the private insurance industry that had proved successful in the United States, the College of Physicians and Surgeons of Saskatchewan, together with the Canadian Medical Association, launched its first offensive during the 1960 provincial election. While the opposition parties, sensing the popularity of "free" health care, chose not to come out against Tommy Douglas's plan, those with money and the media made it clear where they stood — with the doctors. More than $100,000 was raised for a public relations campaign — in today's world, the equivalent of nearly $1 million — which was more than any individual party could spend during the election period. Every home in the province received printed material decrying the horrors of socialized medicine. Radio and newspaper ads were also important parts of the propaganda campaign. In addition to this media bombardment, local chambers of commerce and boards of trade got involved, holding public meetings, which featured presentations by leading physicians and others in the community. Doctors who defied their colleagues and came out in favour of medicare were ridiculed and shunned by the rest of the medical profession.

The campaign was ugly, crude, and effective … at first. People were told, among other things, that the government could institute a policy whereby the mentally infirm would be forced to have abortions or be sterilized. After all, hadn't Tommy Douglas come out in favour of this very thing when he wrote his master's thesis on eugenics in 1933 while at McMaster University in Hamilton, Ontario? And what if the government legislated that civil servants — instead of physicians — would be the ones making decisions on who should or shouldn't be committed to a mental hospital? As scare tactics go, these were pretty good — even if they were more than a little over the top. However, voters in Saskatchewan weren't nearly as naive and easily conned as Americans. When the smoke had cleared and the election results were announced on June 8, 1960, the CCF had taken thirty-seven of the fifty-four seats in the legislature, receiving 42 percent of the vote in a four-way race. Not surprisingly, Tommy Douglas and his cabinet interpreted those results as giving their government a strong mandate to move forward and implement the plan.

And then a funny thing happened.

Tommy Douglas lost his focus for a moment, just long enough to have his arm twisted by his federal cousins up in Ottawa. The brand spanking new New Democratic Party needed a leader, and in the autumn of 1961 Douglas, to the surprise of just about no one, took on the challenge. Now, it's easy to play the "What if?" game. "What if such and such had (or hadn't) happened?" But in this case, Douglas's decision really did change the course of history, having a huge and significant influence on how we ended up with our modern health care system. Had he turned down the offer, Premier Douglas likely would have stayed on as leader of the CCF and ensured a less bumpy ride for his government's pro-medicare legislation. Instead, Douglas handed over the reins of power to Woodrow Lloyd, who then proceeded to very nearly drive the medicare bus over the cliff.

Sensing an opening, the leaders of organized medicine in Saskatchewan redoubled their efforts. If they couldn't stop socialized medicine from being introduced in the province, so went the thinking, perhaps they could put up enough resistance that the new premier would opt for a watered-down version of medicare. One where, instead of setting up a publicly funded system, the government would limit its involvement to simply subsidizing existing medical insurance programs — programs that had been established by and were being run by doctors.

With the help of the Saskatchewan Liberal Party, who had lost five elections in a row and who must have felt the 1964 election would be theirs for the taking now that the popular Douglas was out of the way, Saskatchewan's doctors started preparing for round two. Determined not to lose this time out, the doctors recruited as many community leaders as they could. One such anti-medicare advocate, Athol Murray, a priest, commenting on the doctors' strike, proclaimed on a radio program broadcast province-wide, "This thing may break into violence and bloodshed any day now, *and God help us if it doesn't.*" (Italics mine. The quotation is correct. Murray actually said this.) Things got so bad that the Catholic Church stepped in and ordered the priest to make himself scarce until the battle was over. But Athol Murray had nothing on the right-wing movement known as the Keep Our Doctors (KOD) Committee. Like the Tea Party in the United States, which would turn American politics on its head forty years later, the KOD movement attracted the ill-informed and undereducated. The movement's organizers made it crystal clear they were not only against socialized medicine but wanted to rid the province of all forms of socialism.

As often happens with these public campaigns, though, the anti-medicare side overplayed its hand and badly misread public sentiment. Dedicated groups of CCF supporters, trade unionists, health care advocates, and even a few doctors who dared defy their colleagues at great personal expense formed a loose coalition of their own. Suddenly, community clinics began springing up all around the province — clinics that were determined to enter into contracts with those doctors who'd refused to go on strike. Eventually, it was thought, these clinics, by providing the public with an alternative to the fee-for-service brand of medicine most of Saskatchewan's doctors were fighting so hard to preserve, might prove to be so popular with the public they would become the wave of the future. Those responsible for building and staffing these community clinics would soon form groups such as Citizens in Defence of Medicare and Citizens for a Free Press as a way of countering the other side's propaganda campaign.

Public opinion eventually swung in favour of the government, and the College of Physicians and Surgeons called off the strike in exchange for a few minor tweaks, which led to the signing of an accord with Premier Lloyd and his government that would ensure medical insurance would be controlled by the Government of Saskatchewan, compulsory, universal, and as comprehensive as reasonably possible. A victory for the people of the province and for Woodrow Lloyd — or so it appeared at the time. But in the strange way things often happen, Ross Thatcher, leader of the Saskatchewan Liberal Party, managed to skillfully lay the blame for the 1962 doctors' strike at the feet of the premier and, with the help of the right-wing forces who'd fought so hard against the implementation of medicare in the province, defeated the Lloyd government in the provincial election of 1964. Thatcher then turned around and stunned his supporters by promising to make no changes to medicare when he took over as premier, proving once again that politics is nothing if not unpredictable.

So, what's to be learned from the Saskatchewan experiment more than half a century later? Not much, apparently. While Tommy Douglas has been canonized by the pro-medicare forces — the ones who'd have us believe our health care system, as it is currently constituted, *is* in fact sustainable and that the status quo is just fine, thank you very much — I can't help thinking poor Tommy must be rolling in his grave. Because the pro-medicare bunch are wrong. And if he were still alive, the first person who'd point out that they're wrong would be, ironically enough, the former premier of Saskatchewan. For, you see, Tommy Douglas, despite the mountain of propaganda others have built up around him over the past six decades, was *not* a man stuck in the past — an inflexible, unmovable, and thoroughly stubborn man, whose vision of health care was blurred by misguided and thoroughly useless principles.

Truth be told, the version of medicare Tommy Douglas introduced in Saskatchewan back in the early 1960s was not a finished product — not by a long shot. It was a work in progress. Reorganizing how health care was funded in the province was only the first step. Douglas knew that the only way his plan would work was if all of those involved in the delivery of care embraced the concept of illness prevention and health promotion, as well as the extension of care out into the community. In other words, in order for the new system to succeed, the premier needed buy-in, not just from doctors, nurses, pharmacists, and other health care professionals, but also from the public.

And despite what the pro-medicare forces would have you believe, Tommy Douglas *wasn't* against Canadians paying out of their own pockets to help fund medicare. As a matter of fact, he felt it was important the public make some kind of contribution to the cost of their own health care. "I think that there is value in having every family, and every individual, make some individual contribution," he said. "I think it has a psychological value. I think it keeps the public aware of the cost and gives people a sense of personal responsibility. Even if we could finance [medicare] without a per capita tax, I personally would advise against it." Tommy Douglas, the prairie pragmatist, knew what he was talking about. The "if it's free, it's for me" mentality that has grown up around medicare since it was introduced proves that. Without paying their fair share, people will naturally shrug their shoulders and ignore the true cost of trying to sustain Canada's health care system.

Here's something else you probably didn't know about the form of medicare Tommy Douglas delivered to the people of Saskatchewan. The legislation allowed for a parallel private health care system to exist right alongside the one run by the government. People and doctors could choose to "opt out" of the provincial one if they so desired. In addition to this, Saskatchewan's doctors were allowed to determine their own prices, a practice known as "balance billing." The mind-numbing government monopoly that's currently holding us back and stifling innovation didn't exist until the passing of the Canada Health Act in 1984. What Tommy Douglas was in favour of was a guaranteed, affordable health care system that everyone in his province could access. He felt no one should lose their home or have to declare bankruptcy, as often happens in the United States, just because they got sick. However, the premier had no problem letting people pay a little extra if the public system wasn't meeting their needs. In fact, Douglas himself hired private nurses to care for his daughter Shirley so she could stay at home when she came down with the measles, instead of having to be confined to a public hospital.

Something pro-medicare advocate Shirley Douglas seems to have forgotten.

The Hall Commission and the Introduction of Medicare

While all this was going on in Saskatchewan, significant changes vis-à-vis health care were taking place in the rest of the country, as well. In 1948, Paul Martin Sr., in his role as federal minister of national health and welfare for the Mackenzie King government, announced a number of grants that were intended to help the provinces deal with a variety of health care issues, including public and mental health; the treatment of cancer, tuberculosis, and venereal disease; and the prevention of crippling conditions in children. The grants could also be used for training health care professionals, medical research, and the construction of hospitals. Martin, likewise, introduced the Hospital Insurance and Diagnostic Services Act in 1957, which provided money to any province that met certain criteria, to improve health care services for those who lived there, as well as to explore the creation of a health insurance plan in that province.

Before the act could be fully implemented, though, John Diefenbaker's Progressive Conservative Party surprised just about everyone by winning 112 seats, seven more than Louis St. Laurent's Liberals, in the election that year, which gave the Saskatchewan native the right to form the next government. The following year, Diefenbaker and his party scored the largest majority in Canadian electoral history, taking 208 of the 265 seats available. Three years later, Prime Minister Diefenbaker called upon his old friend and law school chum Justice Emmett Hall to chair a Royal Commission on Health Services. Justice Hall, who also hailed from Saskatchewan coincidentally, was given the responsibility to "inquire into and report upon the existing facilities and the future need for health services for the people of Canada, the resources required to provide such services, and to recommend such measures, consistent with the constitutional division of legislative powers in Canada, as the Commissioners believe will ensure that *the best possible health care is available to all Canadians*" (italics in the original). Among other things, the commission was to examine how best to finance Canada's health care system; what training might be required in the future to properly prepare health care professionals for dealing with patients; what the projected costs of running such a system might be, now and in the future; and what might be done to improve the delivery of health care services.

In addition to Emmett Hall, six others were appointed by the prime minister to serve on the royal commission. These were Alice Girard, a registered nurse; Dr. David M. Baltzan; Professor O.J. Firestone; Dr. C.L. Strachan; Dr. Arthur F. Van Wart; and Wallace McCutcheon (who would leave in 1962 when Prime Minister Diefenbaker appointed him to the Senate). The royal commission — it eventually came to be known as the Hall Commission — would hear from hundreds of Canadians during sixty-seven days of public hearings, which were held in all ten provinces, as well as the Yukon.

Justice Hall himself conducted most of the inquiries, carefully questioning witnesses and experts, in hopes of gaining a better understanding of how Canada's patchwork quilt of health care services was — and, in many cases, *wasn't* — working. The jurist was particularly taken aback by the disparity in the quality of health services he found in different parts of the country, in addition to an alarming lack of access, in some places, to many vital services. Not content with merely hearing from hundreds of individual citizens and delegates representing over four hundred organizations, Justice Hall commissioned twenty-six separate research studies and arranged for his group to visit a number of other countries to study how their health care systems worked. When the Hall Commission released its report in 1964 — it was so comprehensive it was issued in two parts — they recommended Canada adopt a model similar to what Tommy Douglas and the CCF had introduced in Saskatchewan. But Justice Hall took it one step further, proposing that schoolchildren and those on welfare should receive free dental care, and that the disadvantaged and elderly should receive free drugs and prescription glasses. As he told reporters after the report had been released, "The only thing more expensive than good health care is no health care."

Reading the Hall Commission's report all these years later provides a fascinating glimpse into what Canada was like back then as our country approached its centennial. Take, for instance, this: "A nation that in 1962 spent $756 million on cigarettes and tobacco and $973 million on alcoholic beverages can afford the programme we recommend which would involve an additional $466 million in 1971." Or how about this: "The unsatisfactory dental health of the nation and particularly of its children must be attended to as soon as personnel can be trained in one of these crash programmes." Or this: "We recognize that the well-being and happiness of the society is simply the sum total of well-being and happiness of its individual members. It is clear that the well-being of a proportion of the population at any given time is seriously curtailed because of mental or physical disease or impairment that, strictly by the laws of chance, could strike any one of us." Or, finally, this: "There is yet another major reason for an expanding public interest in health. It is the growing awareness of the cost to society as a whole of failure to be concerned and to act on behalf of its members. The most dramatic evidence was the rejection rates of armed services recruits in World War II. With the nation in peril, dependent upon its healthy man- and woman-power for survival, the price we were paying for our past lack of adequate health resources and services was glaringly apparent."

The report continues: "We seem, in a sense, to have become 'insurance minded' in that we now believe that an individual family should not have to bear alone the full cost of risks that could happen to any one of us. Accordingly, if the resources of the whole can be used to strengthen the ability of families and individuals to manage and plan for themselves, then they should be so used." Here, we see the beginning of the "social safety net" — or at least the thinking that would lead to it.

Justice Hall and his fellow commissioners took it one step further, though, coming up with a Health Charter for Canadians. The charter proclaimed:

> The achievement of the highest possible health standards for all our people must become a primary objective of national policy and a cohesive factor contributing to national unity, involving individual and community responsibilities and actions. This objective can best be achieved through a comprehensive, universal Health Services Programme for the Canadian people, IMPLEMENTED in accordance with Canada's evolving constitutional arrangements; BASED upon freedom of choice, and upon free and self-governing

professions and institutions; FINANCED through prepay-
ment arrangements; ACCOMPLISHED through the full
co-operation of the general public, the health professions,
voluntary agencies, all political parties, and governments,
federal, provincial and municipal; DIRECTED towards
the most effective use of the nation's health resources to
attain the highest possible levels of physical and mental
well-being.

Did you catch that bit about "national unity"? This is the poison pill,
the seed planted all the way back in 1964 that would produce a tree with
many limbs and deep roots. The hysteria those two words have led to over
the years, when we're talking about medicare, can't be overstated. As someone
who has fought long and hard for a new and better made-in-Canada health
care system, one that is truly innovative and modern and addresses the fiscal
realities every person in this country must deal with, now and in the future,
I'm frankly appalled at those who continually wrap themselves in the flag
and claim to be the only true patriots in Canada. All because they, unlike
me, support the status quo when it comes to health care.

The last paragraph of the Hall Commission's report is both instructive
and frightening. Entitled, simply enough, "The Future," the section sums
up rather eloquently why medicare was doomed from the start to turn
into Canada's most costly social program, one that, if we don't soon act,
will bankrupt the country by 2030. Here's how the commission's report
concludes:

It is obvious, even if no new programmes are adopted,
that gross expenditures on health services will increase
very substantially by 1971 … The population will be 22.6
million by then, an increase of 24 percent over 1961.
Over the same period hospitalization costs alone will
have increased by over 1.3 billion, or by 145 percent, and
Canada is committed to the hospital programme. *No one*
has suggested curtailing or abandoning it. The sum total of
all our proposals is to add to the hospital programme and
to the existing services the personal health services needed

to round out the concept of comprehensive and universal coverage. These additional services will, if implemented, cost an extra $466 million in 1971. That is the price tag which must be affixed to our proposals. We are fully aware that it is a substantial sum. But we are equally aware that the benefits which will flow from such a comprehensive universal health service will be more than worth the price in terms of good health and human happiness.

By the time the commission made its report, Canadians had been forced to suffer through two rather lengthy and divisive election campaigns — the first election taking place on June 18, 1962, the second on April 8, 1963. In 1962, the Progressive Conservatives were able to hold on to power, but less than a year later John Diefenbaker's minority government fell and Lester B. Pearson found himself occupying the prime minister's office, albeit with a still-wobbly minority. Because of the Pearson government's tenuous situation, and because the party was so deeply divided on the issue of health care, it took a while to decide what to do about Justice Hall's report. With the country's doctors still not completely onside, individual MPs were worried that supporting a plan so similar to the one in Saskatchewan might set off protests and doctor strikes nationwide.

Eventually, cooler heads prevailed and the Medical Care Act was introduced by Allan MacEachen, the minister of national health and welfare, on July 12, 1966. The legislation extended the federal government's original cost-sharing agreements, which had been hammered out in the 1940s and 1950s during the Mackenzie King and Diefenbaker years, so that now medical insurance plans covering physician services would be included. Even then, the Liberals got cold feet, delaying implementation of the new law until July 1, 1968.

Eleven years later, in 1979, Emmett Hall was appointed by Prime Minister Pierre Trudeau to once again examine Canada's health care system, as a sort of follow-up to his earlier work in the 1960s. When Justice Hall submitted his completed report in September of 1980, he recommended eliminating extra-billing and opting-out, as he felt that those things, along with user fees, had the potential to seriously affect equal access to health care services for many Canadians. His findings would lead to the introduction, in

1983, of the Canada Health Act, a piece of legislation that would, in effect, prohibit those practices by financially penalizing any province that allowed them to continue.

Now, I realize hindsight is 20/20 and that it's not fair to pass judgment on those who came before us, especially those honourable men and women who sat, alongside Justice Hall, on that royal commission half a century ago and who tried their best to come up with a solution to our health care challenges. But the problem is … they were working on the *wrong* problem. By focusing chiefly on things that were acting as impediments to Canadians' being able to *afford* health care, Justice Hall and his commissioners inadvertently ensured that we ended up with an insurance scheme instead of a health care system. Not only that, but by ignoring things like nutrition, wellness, and prevention, our so-called health care system is, in reality, little more than a *sickness* system. Imagine that instead of taking your car in for regular maintenance, doing things like changing the oil, rotating the tires, and replacing worn-out wipers and spark plugs, you simply waited until something broke down and your car had to be towed to the shop for repairs. That's the kind of health care system we've ended up with. A system where cost is paramount, where we ration care not by the size of your wallet, as they do in the United States, but by the length of a wait-list. A system that is broken and unsustainable because it wasn't built right in the first place. This, unfortunately, is the legacy of Emmett Hall and his royal commission — a good man who asked the wrong questions and ultimately came up with the wrong solutions. (You might be interested to know, by the way, that even his own son, Dr. John Hall, a distinguished pediatric orthopaedic surgeon in Toronto, Ontario, wanted no part of his father's plan, leaving the Hospital for Sick Children, and thereby escaping socialized medicine, in 1971 to become chief of orthopaedic surgery at Boston Children's Hospital.)

As a consultant and political strategist, I see this all the time. Failing to properly identify the problem first inevitably leads to wrong turns and dead ends. Making matters worse, even when a problem is correctly identified, human beings often try to find quick and easy solutions because we feel we don't have the luxury of time to dig deeper and test out our assumptions. Ironically, taking shortcuts only adds to the length of the journey because so much time is wasted having to backtrack after going down blind alleys. Had Justice Hall and his commissioners been able to take a little more time during their deliberations, I believe they likely would have discovered they'd misidentified the problem. Quality health care *is* expensive and *can* cost an individual a great deal of money — there's no argument there. But to focus solely on finding ways to keep Canadians from having to declare bankruptcy or lose their homes should they fall ill was a mistake. Even worse, not allowing Canadians to contribute financially to their health care, while it might have been popular *politically* back in the day, was a recipe for disaster. No wonder so many people think health care is free. Right from the beginning, medicare was designed in such a way to avoid speaking truth to that lie.

Granted, Canadians no longer lose everything just because they get sick or need an operation, but, and it's a big but, nobody is minding the store. Like teenagers in possession of a credit card with no spending limit, people today don't worry about what health care costs or who's footing the bill. As far as most are concerned, socialized medicine means everything is taken care of by the government. Little do they stop to think about who funds all government activities — the taxpayer. So, naturally, the "health care is free" mindset continues to grow, causing problems for provincial treasuries and finance ministers. By insisting upon going down this road, the federal government is bankrupting the provinces. In the province of Ontario, for instance, close to half the annual budget goes to pay for health care services. *Close to half.* That's ludicrous. As former premier Dalton McGuinty once said, "There will come a time when the Ministry of Health is the only ministry we can afford to have, and we still won't be able to afford the Ministry of Health."

For those defenders of the faith who passionately believe the status quo is the only way, and that we mustn't allow innovation or outside-the-box thinking to intrude upon our government-run, state-monopoly, one-tier health care system, I have but one question: "Are you willing to privatize our education system and turn every road into a toll road?" Because the reality is, if we don't soon do something and drastically overhaul medicare, then, as Dalton McGuinty suggested, we won't have any money left to pay for anything else. "The rent is due." "It's time to pay the piper." "You can't cover the cheque you've written on that account." No matter how you say it, the day of reckoning for our health care system is close at hand.

The Canada Health Act

Walter Cronkite, who was referred to as "the most trusted man in America" during the twenty years he anchored the *CBS Evening News*, once said, "America's health care system is neither healthy, caring, nor a system." He was right when he made that comment and he'd be right if he said the same thing today. Health care in the United States is an embarrassment. Plain and simple. However, before you go getting all smug on me, the same thing could just as easily be said about the health care system here in Canada. It's also neither healthy, caring, nor a system. The reasons for this are many but most of the blame should go to the Canada Health Act, introduced by Pierre Trudeau and his Liberal government on December 12, 1983.

The bill, which was brought forth by Monique Bégin, the federal minister of health and welfare, was subtitled, "An Act relating to cash contributions by Canada and relating to criteria and conditions in respect of insured health services and extended health care services." The preamble to the act stated that "continued access to quality health care without financial or other barriers will be critical to maintaining and improving the health and well-being of Canadians," while the primary objective was "to protect, promote and restore the physical and mental well-being of residents of Canada and to facilitate reasonable access to health services without financial or other barriers." The act, which combined and updated two earlier pieces of legislation — the Hospital Insurance and Diagnostic Services Act, 1957, and the Medical Care Act, 1966 — received royal assent on April 1, 1984. Many of us consider this date to be the beginning of the downward spiral medicare currently finds itself in.

Specifically, the Canada Health Act lays out the criteria, as well as the conditions, that provinces and territories must adhere to in order to be eligible for federal transfer payments under the Canada Health Transfer program. These include public administration, comprehensiveness, universality, portability, and accessibility. As well, extra-billing by physicians or dentists for insured health services under the terms of the health care insurance plan of that province or territory were now banned. Likewise, user fees imposed by hospitals or other health care providers for insured health services were also outlawed. Section 13 of the act lists two additional conditions the provinces had to meet in order not to be penalized further from receiving their full allotment of transfer payments from the federal government:

1. The federal minister of health had the right to access specific information with regard to any province's insured and extended health care systems. This information was to be used in the drafting of annual reports by the Department of Health, which would be delivered each year to Parliament, outlining how each province had administered and delivered health care services during the previous twelve months.

2. The provinces were obliged to recognize the federal government's contribution to the funding of both insured health services and extended health services any time a province released a public document or put out advertising or promotional material concerning medicare in that province.

With all the noise and chatter about the Canada Health Act over the years, it's easy to forget the act only deals with how Canada's health care system is *funded*, not how each individual province sets up its system and delivers care. It's also instructive to remember that as a result of the way our country's constitutional powers are divided, adherence to the conditions set out in the Canada Health Act is completely voluntary. In other words, no province or territory is obligated to embrace the act or follow it to the letter. However, the federal government made sure when they drafted the legislation it would contain enough disincentives that every province would eventually find it to their benefit to fall in line and adhere to the criteria and conditions of the Canada Health Act.

Should any province decide not to comply, something that has happened from time to time over the past three-decades-plus since the act became the law of the land, the federal government had the right to withhold all or part of a transfer payment, depending upon how egregious the offence. For instance, section 20 states quite clearly that should a province violate the prohibition on extra-billing or user fees, an amount equal to that collected would be deducted, dollar for dollar, from that province's transfer payment. In 1993, the federal government reduced British Columbia's transfer payments by more than $2 million after it was discovered the province had allowed roughly forty doctors to extra-bill patients over a four-year period.

Three years later, it was Alberta's turn. The province had its transfer payments reduced by more than $3 million because it turned a blind eye when private clinics started charging patients user fees. Newfoundland and Manitoba also suffered government clawbacks — $323,000 for Newfoundland and $2,056,000 for Manitoba — during the late 1990s, for much the same reason as Alberta. Not to be left out, Nova Scotia was similarly dinged for allowing user fees in private clinics. It's important to note, though, that to date all issues regarding non-compliance have been, for the most part, settled through negotiation or discussions between ministers.

• • •

Those are some of the conditions and administrative details. Let's peel back the skin of the onion and take a closer look at the five principles of the Canada Health Act in a little more detail.

Public Administration

Section 8 of the act says that in order to be eligible for health transfer payments from the federal government, all provincial health plans must be administered and operated on a non-profit basis by a public authority appointed or designated by the government of the province; the public authority must be responsible to the provincial government for that administration and operation; and the public authority must be subject to audit of its accounts and financial transactions by such authority as is charged by law with the audit of the accounts of the province. Again, it's important to note that we're talking here about the *funding* of health care, not the delivery of services. This is one of the things the pro-medicare crowd likes to wave around like a flag. The fact is nowhere does it say that health care services can't be privately delivered, or even, I would argue, privately funded.

Comprehensiveness

Section 9 says that provincial plans must cover all insured health services provided by hospitals, medical practitioners or dentists, and where the law of the province also permits, similar or additional services rendered by other health care practitioners. While the act makes clear in section 2 what is meant by insured services, there's been a significant amount of debate over what should or should not be covered today in the twenty-first century. As has been pointed out, the Canada Health Act almost exclusively defines insured services as those delivered either in hospitals or by physicians. But with the shifting of care from hospitals to the community over the past twenty years, along with a growing dependence on home care, there undoubtedly is a need to re-examine these definitions and modernize them so that they better reflect the world as it exists today, not as it was back in the mid-1980s.

Universality

Section 10 states that all insured persons must be covered for insured health services provided for by the plan on uniform terms and conditions. Strangely, the act's definition of insured persons doesn't include those who may be covered by other provincial or federal legislation, such as active members of the Canadian Armed Forces or Royal Canadian Mounted Police, inmates of federal penitentiaries, those covered by provincial workers' compensation plans, and some Indigenous Peoples. It also doesn't include permanent residents or Canadians returning to live in Canada after having resided in other countries, the latter of whom are subject to a waiting period not to exceed three months before being classified as insured persons.

Portability

According to section 11 of the Canada Health Act, provinces must not impose any minimum period or residence, or waiting period, in excess of three months, before residents of the province are eligible for, or entitled to, insured health services. After the waiting period, the new province or territory of residence assumes health care coverage. It's worth noting that portability provisions are subject to interprovincial agreements, as there can be variations from province to province vis-à-vis what is considered an emergency and whether or not the care received is to be paid at "home" province or "host" province rates, which can also vary from one part of the country to another.

Accessibility

Of the many criteria and conditions of the Canada Health Act, perhaps none have caused as much controversy over the years as this one. Section 12 states that each province's insurance plan must provide for insured services on uniform terms and conditions and on a basis that does not impede or preclude, either directly or indirectly whether by charges made to insured persons or otherwise, reasonable access to those services by insured persons. Further, principle five allows for reasonable compensation for all insured services rendered by medical practitioners or dentists, as well as payments to hospitals to cover the cost of providing care to patients. And yet nowhere in the Canada Health Act is either "reasonable access" or "reasonable compensation" defined.

Part of the reason this fifth and final principle has caused so much consternation over the years, in addition to its lack of definitions and generally ambiguous language, is due to the inconsistencies across Canada when it comes to accessibility. Take abortion, for example. Pro-choice advocates have been quick to point out that access to abortion, defined as a medical service, fails to meet four of the five basic principles of the Canada Health Act. This is because abortion clinics, where most procedures are performed, are not funded equally, nor are these services available in all parts of the country.

•••

To understand the inherent weaknesses of the Canada Health Act, and why our country's health care system is failing to live up to any of the principles set out in the act, it might be instructive to stop for a moment and examine some of the crucial differences between today and 1961, when the Hall Commission was first struck, affecting health care spending. After digesting what follows, I believe you'll have a much better understanding of why government is facing an uphill battle trying to fund health care and put the brakes on the runaway train that is patient demand and utilization of services.

Since the early 1960s, Canada's population has more than doubled, rising from 18.2 million in 1961 to 36.6 million in 2017. Meanwhile, per capita spending on health care during that same period has increased more than sixty times — it was less than $100 per person in the early 1960s while it is a whopping $6,604 per person in 2017.

In 1961, 57 percent of health care in Canada was privately funded, while the rest was covered by government. Today, roughly 70 percent of health care is funded by the government, leaving approximately 30 percent to be covered by the private sector. At the same time that government coverage of health costs has been increasing, Canadian life expectancy has also increased. Over the past fifty-plus years, it has risen from sixty-eight (males) and seventy-nine (females) in 1961 to eighty (males) and eighty-four (females) today, while infant mortality rates, considered by many to be a key indicator of how healthy a country's population truly is, have fallen from 27.3 per 1,000 in 1961 to less than 5 per 1,000.

With the rise in life expectancy, there has been an out-of-control growth in chronic disease in the last few years; today, it eats up more than 70 percent of health care costs in Canada.

If one couples all of that with the sobering news that three health care "tsunamis" — diabetes, obesity, and dementia — are waiting, just around the corner, to swamp our health care system, you'll begin to get some idea of the trouble we find ourselves in.

Obviously, given the spiralling costs of Canada's health care system, the status quo simply can't continue to be an option. Whether we amend the Canada Health Act, add some sunset clauses, or just plain scrap it, the time is fast approaching where doing nothing will be the worst course of action possible. In fact, as I've often said, the best way to ensure we end up with the very thing most Canadians say they don't want, a U.S.-style, two-tier health care system, is by leaving things the way they are.

The reality is we simply can't afford "free" health care in this country anymore. It's too damned expensive and it's not even free — keep in mind that those of us who pay taxes provide the funds for the 70 percent of things medicare actually covers, while the other 30 percent either comes out of our pockets or is taken care of by private insurance, typically as part of the compensation package provided for Canadians by their employers.

And yet, even with all the money being poured into our health care system, there's still not enough to fund patient demand. As a result, wait times are getting longer and longer, putting lives at risk and leading to an unconscionable amount of suffering by forcing people to wait mind-boggling amounts of time in order to access care.

In 2017, for instance, a general practitioner practising in Ontario was informed by a neurologist that it would take that specialist four and a half years to see the patient. Four and a half *years*! This is the legacy of the Canada Health Act. By stifling innovation and pretending we have the best health care system in the world, our elected officials and civil servants have made a mockery of the principles of the health care system that they proclaim they will fight to the end to preserve. As one of the judges in the 2004 Chaoulli case said — a case that involved Dr. Jacques Chaoulli and one of his patients challenging the provincial law that prohibited a patient from using private health insurance to pay for publicly insured health care services — "Access to a wait list is not the same as access to care."

No kidding.

And yet, there are still those who think there's nothing wrong with using the Canada Health Act as a sort of protective shield against the sick and infirm. In British Columbia, for example, Dr. Brian Day, former Canadian Medical Association president and long-time medical director of Cambie Surgery Centre, and some patients, have been trying to convince a judge their Charter rights have been violated by the B.C. government. I won't go into details just yet, other than to tell you that Dr. Day's Charter challenge asks the following fundamental question: Why should Canada, in contrast to every other country on earth, refuse to allow its citizens to purchase private insurance to cover physician and hospital services?

During the first six months of the trial, Dr. Day and his group burned through the $2 million they'd raised by asking those who care about health care and our country to donate to the cause, all because the government had deep pockets and endless resources designed to distract the judge from the real issue and tie up proceedings for months on end. Shamefully, the British Columbia government assigned twenty lawyers to the case and spent $20 million in the first six *months* in hopes that Dr. Day and his patients would run out of money and have to abandon their Charter challenge. Think about that for a moment. A provincial government spent $20 million of our tax dollars in order to ensure our fellow Canadians would be forced to continue to suffer and ultimately die on wait-lists — all in order to prop up the Canada Health Act and maintain the illusion that everything is fine. If that doesn't infuriate you, you'd better check to see if you're still breathing.

And just what is at stake here? What are they fighting about? "Privatization" … "the elephant in the room." The thirteen-letter word that gets everyone, supporters of the status quo and critics, like me, of our non-healthy non-caring health care system, so fired up. As you may or may not know, privatization involves governments — any government, but in Canada most often provincial or territorial governments — shifting responsibilities to the private sector. It's important to remember, as I alluded to earlier, that privatization of financing is not the same as privatization of delivery. Privatization of financing occurs when the government does things like delist services, or cut programs, or reduce fees in such a way as to make it unprofitable for medical practitioners or institutions to continue to offer a particular service.

Privatizing the delivery of health care services is different. There are plenty of examples of this. In many cases, provincial and territorial governments have entered into agreements with the private sector to provide services in non-traditional, noninstitutional settings that are paid for by the government out of public money — typically with an eye toward reducing wait-lists for a politically sensitive constituency, such as seniors (hence the special attention paid to things like cataract surgery and hip and joint replacement, often in the months leading up to an election).

But the privatization of delivery outside the medicare system ... well now, for some reason, that's different. At least it is in the minds of our elected officials and pro-medicare types. "We must not allow two-tier medicine to gain a foothold here in Canada," they say. "It's against everything we believe in as Canadians." Oh, give me a break. What our leaders and those defenders of the status quo — particularly unions — are really concerned about is that the private sector just might deliver a better product at a cheaper price, all because of a little *competition*. But no, no, no ... we can't possibly allow that. It's un-Canadian!

Of course, politicians being politicians, what they truly want is to have it both ways. They acknowledge privately that medicare is indeed unsustainable, and if we don't soon wake up and smell the coffee, we'll end up bankrupting the whole damned country. But they sure as hell don't want to take the blame for allowing a parallel private health care system — what is referred to as the "hybrid solution" — to finally see the light of day and operate (legally) here in Canada. Crazy, isn't it? The fear of stepping on the so-called third rail of Canadian politics, and thereby ending their political careers, has rendered just about every single one of them impotent. But it's not just this that infuriates me. I've been told by a reliable source that the Ontario health ministry has actually commissioned a bunch of reports, trying to figure out a way the government can bring in a hybrid health care system without catching flak.

Perhaps the best way I can illustrate what's wrong with the Canada Health Act and the crazy, mixed-up world it's spawned is by sharing with you a conversation that occurred between Prime Minister Pierre Trudeau and Monique Bégin shortly before the bill became law (an anecdote related by Roy Romanow, the former premier of Saskatchewan and chair of the 2002 royal commission on health care).

One day, the health minister burst into Trudeau's office and said, "I think we have a problem with the legislation. The provinces hate it. The Canadian Medical Association hates it. The hospitals hate it. The opposition hates it."

The prime minister replied, "Where do the people stand?"

"Oh," Bégin replied, "the people love it."

"Well, then, Monique," Trudeau smiled, "what's the problem?"

Thirty-plus years later, the "problem" has become only too obvious.

The Savings and Restructuring Act

It might come as something of a surprise that I've chosen to examine in some detail Progressive Conservative premier Mike Harris's controversial omnibus bill, the Savings and Restructuring Act (which was introduced by Finance Minister Ernie Eves on November 29, 1995), instead of taking a look at Alberta premier Ralph Klein's Health Care Protection Act (which was tabled in the Alberta legislature in the spring of 2000 and appeared to open the door for a parallel private health care system, what Klein would come to refer to as "the third way"), or discussing the impact of NDP premier Bob Rae's decision in the early 1990s to cut medical school enrolment by 10 percent. While both of these are well worth exploring, I feel Harris's omnibus bill had a more significant impact on Ontario's — and, by extension, Canada's — health care system. Not so much because of what was in the bill — and believe me, there was plenty, as dozens of acts were amended and three new ones were introduced over the bill's seventeen schedules — but because it represented something of a missed opportunity.

To understand what I mean by this, go all the way back to the summer of 1990, when Liberal premier David Peterson made a miscalculation for the ages. Worried that the economy, which in the early part of 1990 was beginning to show signs of instability, might collapse just before the next election was scheduled, Peterson called a snap summertime election three years into his mandate, in hopes of catching the opposition parties off guard and taking advantage of a sleepy electorate.

Much to everyone's surprise, the NDP won 74 of the 130 seats when the votes were counted on September 6, 1990, despite capturing only 37.6 percent of the popular vote. New premier Bob Rae stated publicly, once he was sworn in, that even though little more than a third of Ontarians had supported the NDP, he was going to govern as if everyone had voted for his party. This, ultimately, was what would sink Rae and his New Democratic government four and a half years later, as he managed to alienate not only those who had voted for the NDP but also members of the business community and many middle-class voters, who by then felt his government had badly mishandled the economy.

By the time 1995 rolled around, the Ontario Liberal Party had a new leader. Although not a household name, nor a particularly dynamic campaigner, Lyn McLeod was poised to become the next premier of Ontario, according to the polls. As for the Progressive Conservative Party ... well, they and their leader, Mike Harris, were flying well below everyone's radar. They were mired in third place, still struggling to gain traction after the disastrous 1990 campaign, and nobody gave them a ghost of a chance of winning the next election.

But something happened on the way to Lyn McLeod's coronation.

Mike Harris caught a big blue wave. Riding the crest of voter discontent and taking advantage of a bitter and uneasy electorate who'd been battered and bruised by the recession of the early 1990s, the PC leader got everyone's attention by releasing a document calling for a revolution — a *common sense* revolution. Quite possibly the most brilliant piece of campaign literature ever to make its way onto the Canadian political landscape, the *Common Sense Revolution* (CSR) laid out the plan — one that was fully costed and verified by an independent third party — of how Harris and his fellow Conservatives were going to fix what was broken. Tax cuts, welfare reform, the elimination of red tape. It was a bold plan, which most political pundits failed to take seriously. Many thought it was too radical for a middle-of-the-road place like Ontario. Still others thought that while the plan might be viable, there was no way Harris — or, indeed, *any* Canadian politician — would ever go so far as to actually implement these crazy ideas. Boot camps for youth, and chain gangs? Here? No way, the thinking went. Ontarians had no appetite for the man who was fast becoming known to his enemies as the "Newt of the North," after the American speaker of the house Newt Gingrich, who, along with dozens of other Republicans, had ridden their *Contract with America* — a precursor to Harris's *Common Sense Revolution* — to victory in the 1994 U.S. mid-term elections.

Following the televised leaders' debate, however, which many felt Harris had won, the polls started to swing in the PCs' favour. When the votes were tallied on June 8, 1995, the Progressive Conservative Party had captured 82 of the 130 seats and a remarkable 44.8 percent of the popular vote. Mike Harris had just done the impossible, going from third place to first in less than two months, and winning an election that most everyone said he had no business even contesting.

Common sense was back and Ontario would never be the same.

To launch the "revolution" in earnest, though, an impressive first salvo was needed — and the Savings and Restructuring Act was it. From the moment it was read in the legislature by Ernie Eves, Harris's omnibus bill created controversy and generated a whole lot of commentary. The opposition parties cried foul, claiming that the government couldn't cram all those amendments to so many statutes into one bill, to mention nothing of the three new acts the government intended to make part of the bill. After all, omnibus bills were most commonly used for housekeeping matters, not substantive policy reforms. What the Harris government was proposing was unprecedented as far as the opposition parties were concerned.

Debate raged on and on for days. Insults were flung across the aisles of the Ontario legislature during question period. Outside, protesters held up their signs and chanted their slogans, while the OPP riot squad waited patiently, batons and shields at the ready. Everyone expected the speaker of the house, long-time PC MPP Al McLean, would rule the bill out of order, thereby forcing the government back to the drawing board where they'd have to break the behemoth into smaller, easier-to-swallow pieces of legislation. But McLean dropped the ball, something he would do frequently during his short tenure as speaker, and ruled in the government's favour.

To understand the scope of what was being proposed here, one need only closely examine the heft of this particular piece of legislation. As alluded to earlier, the Savings and Restructuring Act contained seventeen schedules, amended forty-four separate statutes, created three new acts, and repealed two others, all while granting frightening new powers to a number of cabinet ministers. Small wonder people were soon referring to it as the "bully bill." When first introduced, the bill contained some two hundred pages and landed on each parliamentarian's desk with a rather noticeable thud. Once passed, it would allow the Harris government to tell doctors where they could and couldn't practise; close hospitals on the advice of the soon-to-be-constituted Health Services Restructuring Commission, which would be chaired by Duncan Sinclair; force the Ontario public service to accept mandatory binding arbitration; turn Ontario highways into toll roads; and compel certain Ontario municipalities to amalgamate. It was a courageous plan, a course of action that would change the political landscape of the province for years to come — although the government's critics suggested it would more likely scorch the earth than bring about change in a thoughtful, civilized manner. The premier wanted the bill passed as quickly as possible, preferably before the legislature rose for the Christmas break, and scheduled three days of committee hearings in Toronto in December for those opposing the bill to have their say.

The CSR train was about to leave the station ... until someone noticed that little-known Liberal backbencher Alvin Curling was standing on the tracks, blocking the way.

Curling, who would sit in the speaker's chair himself after Dalton McGuinty became premier in 2003, caused an uproar by refusing to vote on a routine motion. Speaker McLean, as required by parliamentary rules, ordered Curling to be removed from the chamber. When the sergeant-at-arms arrived at the Liberal MPP's seat to escort him out, other opposition members surrounded Curling, linking arms so no one could touch him. McLean, befuddled, gave up and left the chamber instead, plunging the House into a kind of "suspended animation." Long story short, Curling spent the rest of the day and all of the night in his chair, emerging the following morning — but only after the government had given in and agreed to hold province-wide committee hearings after Christmas.

If you've never had the pleasure of attending a legislative committee hearing in person, or even of catching a few minutes of one on TV, let me take a moment here to share my experience. I had, by this time, been an employee of the Ontario Medical Association for roughly eight months.

Dr. Albert Schumacher, the chair of the OMA's political action committee, and CEO David Pattenden had convinced the rest of the board of directors it was important for the association to "show the flag" at every one of the hearings. So I — along with fellow OMA staffers Camille Sobrian and Sandra Wismer, as well as various board members — was ordered to criss-cross the province for two weeks in January in hopes of, if not actually derailing the bill, at least slowing it down a little. Like the classic Steve Martin movie, with me playing John Candy's role, we covered eleven cities in ten days, riding every combination of "trains, planes and automobiles" imaginable.

To the best of my memory, the festivities kicked off on Monday, January 8, 1996, in Timmins, Ontario. The woman at the front desk of the hotel we'd checked into warned us to be careful venturing outside, as the temperature that night was predicted to go as low as -30° Celsius — without factoring in the wind chill. Having never experienced such temperatures before, I stepped out the front door of the hotel later that evening and immediately felt my nasal hairs turn to ice. Clearly, I wasn't in Kansas anymore. Once the first day of hearings wrapped up less than twenty-four hours later, we boarded a Bearskin Airlines flight and flew to the next location. After Timmins, it was some combination of Thunder Bay, Sudbury, Ottawa, Kingston, and Peterborough. I returned home on Saturday, took care of my laundry and recharged my batteries as best I could, before taking the train — along with Camille and Sandra — to Windsor, Ontario, on January 14 in order to help our local OMA members prepare their presentations for the next day. Once the committee had heard from everyone who was scheduled to appear before them, we hopped in a rental car and began working our way back to Toronto via London, Kitchener-Waterloo, Niagara Falls, and Hamilton.

Following days of tears, tantrums, and testimony, the government finally buckled and announced on that final Thursday they would be making public a significant number of amendments to their own bill just before the last day of hearings got under way in Hamilton on Friday, January 19, 1996. We arrived in the Steel City around four-thirty that afternoon, having taken the QEW from Niagara Falls. Sandra announced she was going for a swim in the hotel pool, while Camille and I went back to our rooms to check in with OMA headquarters in Toronto. Shortly after the three of us finished eating dinner, around eight p.m., I ran into the health minister's policy advisor and managed to convince him to hand over the government's amendments so I could see what they'd come up with, telling him I'd return them to his hotel room in an hour. Instead of reviewing the amendments myself, I quickly had the front desk fax them back to Toronto, where OMA board member and chief negotiator Dr. Bill Orovan was eagerly waiting to receive them. Once I'd confirmed the amendments had arrived safe and sound, I returned the original package to the minister's advisor, as promised, and went to bed.

Dr. Orovan was first up the next morning and wasted no time letting the government representatives at the hearing know what he thought of their amendments. In a calm, measured voice, the good doctor gave the government members of the committee — including future finance minister Janet Ecker and future health minister Tony Clement — a blunt, to-the-point lecture on how they'd screwed up and got everything wrong. Standing at the back of the room, I couldn't help noticing that both Ecker and Clement were looking at me — as was the minister's policy advisor, whose eyes looked like they were about to pop out of his head — with steam coming out of their collective ears. Once Dr. Orovan finished his testimony, members from all three parties on the committee took turns asking him questions. Ten minutes later, committee chair Jack Carroll called for a short recess, and everyone stood up to stretch their legs and grab a coffee. I pulled the schedule out of my coat pocket to see which organization was up next, when I suddenly became aware of something heading my way — something that felt a lot like a freight train. I looked up just in time to see the aforementioned Janet Ecker coming at me, full force. She body-slammed me against the wall and asked what the hell was going on. The government, she informed me, had gone to great lengths to amend the bill in such a manner that would make doctors happy. And now Dr. Orovan had gone and crapped all over it.

Interestingly enough, this was not the first time I'd been body-slammed by a common sense revolutionary. Two months earlier, Paul Rhodes, a senior advisor to Premier Harris and a former government relations manager with the Ontario Medical Association, had taken it upon himself to bounce me off the wall in a room at the Hamilton Convention Centre.

On that occasion Dr. Schumacher and I had taken another rental car and driven to the PC Party's convention right after the OMA's November council meeting, at which the council had voted *not* to invoke the Rand formula on their members. (The Rand formula had been named after Justice Ivan Rand, who in 1946 declared that those who benefited from a union or association's activities were duty bound to pay mandatory dues, whether they wanted to be a member of said union or association or not.) The OMA council felt it wouldn't be right to collect dues when the Harris government was planning to strip the OMA of its representation rights. Rhodes apparently had told Harris the OMA would never give up Rand and all those guaranteed millions of dollars in membership dues, which is why the premier had decided to go ahead and include the line about representation rights in the original version of the *Savings and Restructuring Act* … but then, the OMA did exactly what Rhodes predicted they wouldn't do. Hence body-slam number one, delivered by Paul Rhodes. Which, as mentioned, was followed by body-slam number two, delivered by Janet Ecker two months later.

Who knew politics could be such a contact sport? I was learning fast.

At the beginning of this segment, I suggested that the *Savings and Restructuring Act* represented something of a missed opportunity. While it's true that the mother of all omnibus bills did create the legislative framework for the much-needed restructuring of Ontario's hospital system, as well as setting in motion the amalgamation of various municipalities throughout the province, which would ultimately lead to, among other things, the creation of the "megacity" now known as Toronto, the bill could have done so much more. Had Mike Harris been a true revolutionary, he would have seized upon this opportunity — this rare moment in time when all the stars appeared to finally be in alignment — to introduce a parallel private health care system. After all, Harris had been handed a strong mandate from the people of Ontario six months earlier. And he wouldn't have to go to the polls and face the electorate for another three or four years. True, some were protesting rather vehemently the changes Harris was making, but for the most part, their shenanigans did more harm than good to their causes and only increased the general public's support for the government. Plainly, Ontarians had bought into Harris's "tough love" approach.

Another reason I believe Premier Harris would've succeeded had he had the courage to make the hybrid solution a part of the *Savings and Restructuring Act* has to do with the fascinating political science experiment he and his advisors decided to conduct in the late 1990s.

Let me explain.

Traditionally, when political parties contest an election, they "narrow-cast" — in other words, they aim their message and spend the vast majority of their time and resources on those who either will or might vote for them. Rule of thumb says that one-third of voters will vote for any given party, one-third will not, and one-third might, if they knew a little more about the party and, especially, its local candidate. As a result, strategists set things up so that candidates pretty much ignore the one-third who won't vote for them, while concentrating mainly on those who will definitely vote for them and those who might do so. This is how you put together a winning coalition in electoral politics.

Once you're elected, however, and form a government, you typically do what Bob Rae did in 1990 and "broadcast" — you govern not just for those who elected you, but for everyone. What made Mike Harris's revolution so unique is that for the first time in Canadian political history, a party that was elected by narrowcasting actually *governed* the same way. Harris and his team didn't care about the 55 percent who hadn't voted Progressive Conservative in the 1995 Ontario election. He governed for the 45 percent that did. And guess what? It worked. Four years later, in 1999, Harris won his second consecutive majority government by capturing — wait for it! — 45.1 percent of the popular vote.

Regrettably, the PC premier squandered this opportunity, as well, and soon lost his way. Two years into his second mandate, Harris announced his resignation and was replaced by former finance minister Ernie Eves. Unfortunately, Eves proved to be something of a disappointment. Voters came to see him as little more than "Harris lite," and when the next election took place they voted for Dalton McGuinty — a real liberal — preferring his policies to Eves's "red tory" brand of liberalism. Although some would say the revolution died along with Mike Harris's political career, the final nail in the coffin came on October 2, 2003, when Dalton McGuinty's Liberals captured 46.4 percent of the popular vote, winning 72 of 103 seats, setting the table for even more health care missed opportunities in the years to come.

The Commitment to the Future of Medicare Act

Before we continue our journey together and explore the Commitment to the Future of Medicare Act, an especially abhorrent piece of legislation that was introduced by George Smitherman, Premier Dalton McGuinty's health and long-term care minister, on November 27, 2003, I'd like to share a story with you. It's about my dad and about how he would've died had I not refused to accept the status quo and intervened instead. But mostly it's about a bunch of caring, dedicated doctors and the actions they took to help me manipulate the system by putting my special health care knowledge and their contacts to work, in a way that my fellow Canadians could only dream of, in order to save my father's life.

It was around the middle of September 2000. My mother phoned me at work, saying she was worried about my father. He seemed to have lost interest in everything, was sitting in his chair staring at the TV, and was complaining of headaches. I told my mom I'd leave work early and come as soon as I could get away. After hanging up the phone, I rented a car and made the trek to their home, where I discovered — alarmingly — my mother hadn't been exaggerating. My father looked awful. His hair was sticking out everywhere and he hadn't shaved in a week. He was in his seventy-eighth year and fit and trim as a result of spending thirty-three years as a Bell Telephone lineman. But looking at him then, there was obviously something wrong. He looked like a man who'd lost the will to live. This was so not like my father.

After talking with my dad for a few minutes, I slipped away and called one of the OMA board members, Dr. Garnet Maley, at his office. I explained as best I could what was going on with my father. Dr. Maley listened patiently, then instructed me to bundle my dad into the car and drive him straight to the hospital. We were to go to the emergency department and tell them my father was experiencing the "worst headache of his life," which apparently is code for "this patient is on the verge of having a stroke." I thanked the doctor for his advice, got off the phone, and spoke with my mother, who then helped me get my uncharacteristically docile dad into the car. Upon arrival at the hospital in Peterborough, we went inside and told the triage nurse in the emergency department about my father's headache. Within minutes, he saw a doctor and was taken to the X-ray department for a brain scan.

An hour later, after my father had returned, a doctor came by and informed us that my father was a very lucky man. He had not one blood clot but *two* — one on each side of his head. If he'd only had the one, the doctor informed us, it was likely my father would have suffered a major stroke, one that probably would've killed him. Because he had a blood clot on either side of his head, however, they were more or less exerting an equal amount of pressure on his brain — hence the headaches — which was the only thing keeping him from stroking out. Talk about your good news, bad news scenario.

While it was true my father hadn't suffered a stroke — not yet, anyway — he was in danger and needed surgery as soon as possible. And that's when luck proved to be a lady indeed. "Steve!" a voice called out from the hallway behind me. "What are you doing here?" It was one of the doctors I'd trained in the art of political action, back when he was still a resident and we were fighting with the Harris government over the changes they were so hell-bent on implementing with regard to how doctors practised medicine. I explained my father's situation and asked him if he could remember the name of the neurosurgeon who'd moved from Windsor, Ontario, to Etobicoke the previous year. I'd met her during the Savings and Restructuring Act hearings in the winter of 1996, when she'd testified before the legislative committee. "Not only do I remember her name," the doctor informed me, "I just so happen to have her cell number. Let me give her a call and see if she can operate on your father right away."

Not surprisingly, the neurosurgeon remembered me from the hearings and was grateful for my help. Now, it was her turn to help me. She asked me to bring my father and the scan the doctors had taken of his brain and come the following morning to the hospital she worked out of. Fortunately, the next day was a Saturday, so there was little or no traffic as I made my way to the hospital. The neurosurgeon was waiting for us and, after reviewing the aforementioned brain scan, informed me she would be operating on my father first thing the next morning — Sunday, September 24, 2000.

Luckily, my father was a tough old bird, having survived the Great Depression and the Second World War, and came through the surgery with flying colours. We took him home the following weekend, where he would recover with the help of my mom and me. While there, my father and I watched the state funeral for former prime minister Pierre Trudeau, who'd passed away less than a week after my father's brain surgery. As young Justin Trudeau eulogized his father, the irony wasn't lost on either one of us that, had it not been for serendipity, I might be eulogizing my father at the same time.

I tell this story because had the events described occurred four or five years later, after the Commitment to the Future of Medicare Act had been passed into law, both the doctors involved in saving my father's life and I would've been guilty of violating the act and would have put ourselves at risk of being fined up to $25,000. Now, I know what you're thinking. *It's a good thing Dalton McGuinty's government passed such a piece of legislation. It means that people like you are no longer able to take advantage of your connections and work the system in order to get faster treatment and better service.* But you see, that's the problem with medicare. The system promotes mediocrity and punishes innovation. So long as everyone has to wait in line and suffer needlessly, then, as far as our elected officials are concerned, everything is fine. But the truly infuriating part for me is that instead of making decisions based on logic and medical evidence, our leaders continually play politics with our lives. And the Commitment to the Future of Medicare Act is a perfect example of this.

Here's why.

In the autumn of 2003, Premier McGuinty instructed his health minister to come up with a piece of legislation to honour the work of former Saskatchewan premier Roy Romanow, who had been appointed in 2002 — this time by Prime Minister Jean Chrétien — to chair yet another commission looking into Canada's health care system. The Royal Commission on the Future of Health Care in Canada — which produced what's known as the Romanow Report — made forty-seven recommendations, in hopes of ensuring that Canada's health care system would be sustainable long into the future. Romanow's report set the stage for another round of federal-provincial meetings, which would ultimately lead to Paul Martin's investment in 2004 of $41 billion in additional funding over the next ten years through the newly created Canada Health Transfer. "A fix for a generation," Martin called it.

• • •

George Smitherman's remarks, as he testified before the legislative committee looking into the Commitment to the Future of Medicare Act, are particularly enlightening and well worth a second look in light of what Roy Romanow's royal commission had to say about the state of Canada's health care system. "Medicare does need our protection," Smitherman began. Continuing, he said,

There are various forces alive and well in Canada that claim the only way to fix public health care is to abandon its principles and to offer a parallel private system for those who have money. Our government disagrees entirely. In Canada, health care is not a commodity to be bought or sold; it is a basic right. Are changes needed? Absolutely, but the changes we are talking about will bring our public system back to its founding values. These changes will breathe new life into medicare. Real, significant, system-wide change is needed to make medicare more responsive, more focused on quality outcomes and more accountable to the 12 million Ontarians who own the health care system.

Smitherman went on to say that no one had made the case for medicare renewal as passionately and as persuasively as Roy Romanow. "He laid out the challenge ahead this way: 'Canada's journey to nationhood has been a gradual, evolutionary process, a triumph of compassion, collaboration and accommodation, and the result of many steps both simple and bold.... The next step is to build upon this proud legacy and transform medicare into a system that is more responsive, comprehensive and accountable to all Canadians.'" The health minister then said something quite remarkable. "Bill 8 [the Commitment to the Future of Medicare Act] gives us an effective tool to change the status quo in Ontario."

Say what? Change the status quo? If only.

Not content to stop there, Smitherman went on, explaining,

[The Commitment to the Future of Medicare Act] is transformative legislation because it reinforces the principle of the Canada Health Act by strengthening prohibitions against two-tier medicine. [It] requires mandatory reporting of activities like queue-jumping and extra-billing and gives the ministry greater ability to uncover potential instances of extra-billing and queue-jumping. For example, the general manager of OHIP would be able to collect key information from providers if they suspect that payment for queue-jumping has taken place. Today, consumers and providers who witness queue-jumping and extra-billing have no protection against reprisals if they speak up. [The Commitment to the Future of Medicare Act] would protect whistle-blowers who expose two-tier activities because we believe that the people who own the system ought to be involved in helping to defend it.

The health minister then concluded his remarks by giving a shout-out to Roy Romanow himself:

We all have an enormous opportunity to deliver on Roy Romanow's vision. To quote Roy Romanow a few weeks ago at the RNAO annual general meeting, "Ontario's [Commitment to the Future of Medicare Act] has some very important features that reinforce what we had in mind regarding accountability. It seems to me that Ontario wants to do the 'real work' required to ensure medicare sustainability" … I'll close on this point, because I do believe this is work that has been inspired by the work that Roy Romanow did on behalf of our country and I'm very proud to have his comment be the last one as relates to my opening remarks.

Elizabeth Witmer, who'd served as health minister under Mike Harris in the late 1990s, was the first opposition member to comment on what George Smitherman had to say. "My question to the minister would be," Witmer began, "you talk about two-tier, and you talk about the fact that this bill is going to eliminate queue-jumping or extra-billing. I would suggest to you that the key problem is the fact that the reason we have two-tier, the reason people queue-jump, the reason people do this is because the waiting lists are too long. And I guess one of the things I don't see addressed in this bill at all is the whole issue of waiting lists or an improvement in the access to care."

Responding, the health minister said, "I don't think it's very helpful or healthy to have the debate about [this bill] turned into a discussion about everything a person might want in health care."

Oh, really?

Smitherman went on to say, "Wait times are a critical focus of our government. We're increasingly results-based."

History would prove him wrong on that one. Perhaps we can chalk it up to what Premier Kathleen Wynne would later describe as a "stretch" goal.

"My final point to you," the health minister said, wrapping up his response to Elizabeth Witmer,

> to go back to what you said with respect to waiting lists, is we don't even have a mechanism for proper capturing of wait-time challenges as they exist on a region-by-region basis. I think you know that from your days as minister. But our drive toward that is really an essential ingredient in the Ontario Health Quality Council. I think that Romanow sees progress in [the Commitment to the Future of Medicare Act], but I'm not here to suggest to you that the bill is the be-all and end-all for what our government is about but an important framing for much of what we intend to do.

Witmer's response to Smitherman was nothing short of brilliant. "Thank you very much, Minister," she said. "On the issue of accountability, I guess one of the complaints we've heard over and over from presenters is the fact that this bill does not hold you accountable for your actions. Instead, it does bestow some tremendous power. I guess one of the questions I would ask, and I know it was a concern for the stakeholders, is why is accountability only a one-way street in this bill, if it's such a key principle of medicare? The accountability is only on the health care provider group; it's not on the ministry or the minister."

Touché.

With the passing of the Commitment to the Future of Medicare Act, the Liberal government's so-called Transformation Agenda could now get under way in earnest. Ill-conceived, totally irrational, and punitive in nature, it caused more damage in Ontario than even Bob Rae's mishandling of the recession in the early 1990s. Even worse, other provinces, including British Columbia and Alberta, soon began to make changes to their health care systems based in no small part on what Ontario — led by George Smitherman, the Transformation Agenda's chief architect and head cheerleader — had come up with. Nicknamed "Furious George" because of his propensity for knocking heads and locking horns with those who disagreed with him, Smitherman might well have gone down in history as the worst minister of health Ontario has ever dealt with ... had it not been for those who came after him.

First, there was David Caplan — son of former David Peterson–era health minister Elinor Caplan. His tenure was brief — less than two years — as he was forced to walk the plank after the Liberal government's eHealth fiasco (more on that later). Then came Deb Matthews — Peterson's sister-in-law — who managed to last five years before being promoted to the newly created position of chair of the treasury board after the 2014 election. An early supporter of Kathleen Wynne, Matthews somehow managed to survive the Ornge air ambulance scandal — an affair that included allegations of sexual improprieties, possible misappropriation of funds, and inappropriate use of taxpayer dollars to fund MBA courses for senior staff — that brought howls from the opposition parties, as well as calls for her resignation, after she admitted she hadn't read a report detailing the frankly troubling leadership of Ornge's founder, Dr. Chris Mazza. She hung on long enough, however, to seriously poison the relationship between Ontario's doctors and the province, making thirty-seven arbitrary changes to the OHIP fee schedule — targeting hundreds of services provided by cardiologists, ophthalmologists, and radiologists — in hopes of saving $338 million.

All of which paved the way for Dr. Eric Hoskins.

Hoskins, who, along with his wife, Dr. Samantha Nutt, had run an organization called War Child Canada before entering politics in 2009, was appointed minister of health and long-term care by Premier Wynne in 2014, after he had broken his promise to support Sandra Pupatello and crossed the floor to join Kathleen Wynne's team during the Ontario Liberal leadership convention the previous year. A medical doctor by training, Dr. Hoskins was thought by many to be an inspired choice for health minister, especially after the premier named another physician, Dr. Robert Bell, Hoskins's deputy minister. After all, went the thinking, how could Ontario's doctors possibly complain when one of their own had not only been appointed minister of health but another had been appointed the deputy? Unfortunately for Ontario's doctors, Dr. Hoskins proved to be no friend of physicians. Finishing the work that George Smitherman had started with the Commitment to the Future of Medicare Act and that Deb Matthews had continued with the implementation of the Transformation Agenda, Hoskins showed his true colours by attacking his colleagues at every turn, accusing them of bilking the system and putting their own financial interests ahead of those of their patients.

By the time the minister got around to introducing his own draconian pieces of legislation — the Patients First Act and the Protecting Patients Act — in 2016 and 2017 respectively, Dr. Hoskins had done what seemed impossible to most observers, wrestling away the title of "worst health minister" ever from Deb Matthews, who'd earlier taken the title from George Smitherman. If you wanted to put the needs of patients *last* while putting their lives at risk, you couldn't have figured out a better way to do it than by bringing forth the Patients First Act and the Protecting Patients Act.

After fifteen years in power, the Ontario Liberals' work was complete. They'd succeeded in transforming the province's health care system. Sadly, not for the better.

PART II

"IF IT'S FREE, IT'S FOR ME"

I was born on December 31, 1958. A Wednesday. Legend has it I came into the world at seven o'clock in the morning, which just happened to be when the night shift was ready to call it a day and the day shift was poised to take over. My mom, who had finally gone into labour several hours after having been driven to the hospital by my father the night before, told me years later that one of the nurses, anxious to go home, said, "She can wait," while another one — perhaps a little closer to the action — exclaimed, "No, she can't!" My first act, shortly after the doctor spanked me into life, was to piss all over everyone.

Funny how some things never change.

I wish I could tell you a momentous, unforgettable event happened that day or that I share a birthday with someone famous. Sir Anthony Hopkins — of Hannibal Lecter fame — was born on December 31, 1937. Eleven years later — December 31, 1948 — Buffalo Sabres' sniper René Robert, a member of the famed French Connection line along with Gilbert Perreault and Rick Martin, was also born on New Year's Eve. Other than American actor Val Kilmer, who made his first appearance one year after me — on December 31, 1959 — that's pretty much it. For those who follow sports closely, the New York Yankees once again won the World Series in 1958, defeating Hank Aaron and the Milwaukee Braves four games to three, while the Montreal Canadiens were on their way to winning a fourth consecutive Stanley Cup. The Winnipeg Blue Bombers defeated the Hamilton Tiger-Cats to capture the 1958 Grey Cup. And the Baltimore Colts, led by a young Johnny Unitas, defeated the New York Giants, 23–17, to emerge victorious in the NFL's first-ever sudden-death overtime game — a contest many refer to as "The Greatest Game Ever Played."

So, what's all this got to do with the price of tea in China? Well, quite simply, if you remember any of these things, then you — like me — are likely a boomer, possibly even a zoomer. Boomers are the generation who were born following the Second World War — typically defined as those born between 1946 and 1964, although some have it as being between 1946 and 1965. Zoomers are boomers that go the extra mile. They are health-conscious people — some would say health "nuts" — who exercise every day, pay attention to their dietary needs, and calculate their daily nutritional intake based upon variables such as age, gender, and weight. Bottom line: they're people who live their lives to the fullest and intend to keep on doing so for as long as possible.

Whether you're a boomer or a zoomer, however, doesn't much matter; you're part of the largest demographic in Canada — a demographic that is, obviously, entering its senior years. And the fact is we're about to see the biggest demographic shift in our nation's history, according to Statistics Canada. Take the year 2015, for example. It marked the first time that Canada had more people over the age of sixty-five than under fifteen. Those in the fifty to sixty-nine age group made up 27 percent of the general population, compared with just 18 percent two decades ago. Even more astonishing, the number of people over sixty-five years of age represented 16 percent of the population — more than double the percentage in 1971.

The effect on our health care system of these demographic shifts will be huge. For one thing, we'll have more people living longer, richer lives than ever before. Unfortunately, no matter how good a job people do of taking care of themselves, various body parts will inevitably begin to wear out and the person's general health will also begin to break down. Imagine a world, if you will, in which those in their eighties and nineties are having hip replacement surgeries, heart and lung transplants, and even Botox injections and facelifts — all in order to look more youthful and keep up with the younger generations. Along with an increase in the number of surgeries required to repair the failing bodies of the elderly, we will soon see an unprecedented increase in pharmaceutical use. Not only will people in their "golden years" be ingesting great gobs of pills to control their high blood pressure and cholesterol levels, who's to say they won't also be demanding that medicare cover Viagra and Cialis to help extend their love lives?

Who will provide all of the services needed to treat the massive numbers of seniors? More importantly, where will all the money come from to pay for everything? That's the bigger question. How will Canada deal with the financial strain all those seniors will place on its health care system? Remember, not only will Canadians be accessing health care services in greater and greater numbers than ever before, the vast majority will also be retiring or — at the very least — drastically reducing their workloads. This means that at the precise moment we'll require more tax dollars to help fund all this extra health care, there'll be fewer workers around to help pay for it through their taxes. And while increased immigration, coupled with a raising of the retirement age to, say, seventy or seventy-two years of age, could offer some relief, the fact is Canada has a significant math problem — there just aren't going to be enough people working to pay for their health care needs and those of their parents and aunts and uncles, who've retired but still have many years to go before they're pushing up the daisies. Add to this the cost of new treatments and technologies, along with the greying of our medical professionals — in the province of Ontario alone, it's thought that 20 to 30 percent of doctors will retire within the next two or three years — and it becomes apparent that if we don't soon start thinking outside the box, then we're going to find ourselves boxed in, and facing a bleak future indeed.

This is why, on this part of our journey, I'm going to take a look at some things you might not have thought about — at least when it comes to understanding why Canada's health care system was designed the way it was and why it's failing us so badly: the myth of "free" health care; the "third rail"; an insurance scheme, not a system; nutrition, wellness, and prevention: the flip side of sickness; finding a family doctor and dealing with wait-lists; eyes and teeth versus pharmacare; Dr. Google; "Cancer Inc."; medical assistance in dying; and three health care tsunamis: obesity, diabetes, and dementia.

The Myth of "Free" Health Care

On February 17, 2002, the eleventh episode of *The Simpsons'* thirteenth season aired on the Fox network. Entitled "The Bart Wants What It Wants," it revolved around Bart Simpson's infatuation with actor Rainier Wolfcastle's daughter, Greta, whom he met at a private-school fair. The "plot" — if an episode of *The Simpsons* can ever be said to truly have a plot — pretty much goes like this: Boy wins girl. Boy loses girl. Boy travels to Canada in order to win her back, after his best friend — Milhouse, of course — accompanies Greta to the Great White North, where her father is shooting a movie.

Along the way, the Simpson family makes a brief stopover in Toronto. Stepping off the bus, Bart's mother, Marge, exclaims, "It's so clean and bland … I'm home!"

Bart's father, Homer, oblivious as always, walks straight into traffic, ignoring a DON'T WALK sign, telling his daughter Lisa not to worry because Canada has free health care. Not surprisingly, a car knocks Homer ass over teakettle. "I'm rich!" he cries out, flying through the air.

Five years later, on May 19, 2007, *Sicko*, a documentary by American filmmaker Michael Moore, premiered at the Cannes Film Festival. The film purports to be an investigation of the American health care industry, focusing specifically on how health insurance works in the United States, as well as the role played by Big Pharma. Moore compares the for-profit, non-universal U.S. health care system with non-profit, universal systems in Canada, the United Kingdom, France, and Cuba … and finds his country's system wanting. An interesting film, perhaps, but for the purposes of this discussion the part that's really fascinating involves the segments shot in Canada. In one of these, a Canadian citizen talks about Tommy Douglas, who, he informs Moore, was voted the "Greatest Canadian" in a 2004 poll for his contributions to Canada's health care system. The filmmaker also interviews a surgeon while in our country and spends some time speaking with patients waiting in the emergency department of one of Canada's publicly funded hospitals.

While *Sicko* generally received positive reviews, some critics — such as consumer advocate John Stossel — complained that Moore had played "fast and loose" with the facts. Writing in an article that appeared in the *Wall Street Journal*, Stossel stated that Julie Pierce's husband, Tracy, who lived with Julie in Kansas City, Missouri, and was featured in the documentary, would likely not have been saved by the bone marrow transplant his health insurer denied him. Stossel then went on to point out that the treatment the Pierces were hoping Tracy would receive, in all probability, would not have been available in a universal health care system either, as a result of long wait-lists and other forms of rationing in countries such as Canada and the United Kingdom. In an article published in the *New Yorker*, journalist Michael C. Moynihan called *Sicko* "touching, naive and maddeningly mendacious, a clumsy piece of agitprop that will likely have little lasting effect on the health care debate." In yet another piece, film critic and former editor of *Rolling Stone* magazine Kurt Loder called out Moore for "cherry-picking the facts, manipulating interviews, and building his film around unsubstantiated assertions." While the U.S. health care system undoubtedly needs reform, Loder admitted, he felt Moore's advocacy for increased government control was not the way to go, as many services currently under the control of the American government are neither cost effective nor particularly efficient.

The world is, without a doubt, enamoured with Canada's health care system and the "free" health care we offer to our citizens. But is health care, as it's currently set up here in Canada, truly free? A 2017 report by the Fraser Institute suggests Canadian health care is anything but free. Using the same proprietary system researchers at the institute use to calculate their "Tax Freedom Day," here's what the Fraser Institute came up with. The average Canadian family — consisting of two adults and two children and earning about $127,000 per annum — will pay roughly $12,000 a year for health care in Canada. While some might think that's a bargain, the Fraser Institute disagrees. Out-of-control health care costs are growing at an alarming rate, the researchers say — 173 percent over the last twenty years, compared with things like food (54.6 percent) and shelter (93.4 percent). And while critics, like economist Richard Shillington, for instance, claim the institute's definition of an "average" Canadian based on income earned or income tax paid is nowhere near what a typical Canadian makes and pays, Bacchus Barua, one of the authors of the study, defended the findings, reminding everyone that the value of such a study lies in making Canadians aware that public health care is not free. "If you ask the average person," Barua said, "I think many would struggle to give you an answer for how much they paid for public health care last year or what they can expect to pay going forward."

No kidding.

One thing I know for sure is that Canada's free health care system is damned expensive. Don't believe me? Let's turn to the Canadian Institute for Health Information (or CIHI, as the institute is more generally referred to) and see what kind of story its numbers tell us. CIHI was created in 1994 as a non-profit, independent organization dedicated to forging a common approach to Canadian health information. The institute provides comparable and valuable data and information that are meant to be used to improve health care system performance and population health across the country. As a result, stakeholders working with CIHI are able to utilize its databases, evidence-based reports, and other forms of analysis in developing their own individual decision-making processes. The institute ensures that the privacy of all Canadians is protected by guarding the confidentiality of all personal health information used in creating their databases and reports.

As mentioned elsewhere, Canada currently spends more than $200 billion a year on health care. That's a lot of money, no matter how you slice it. So, what are all those health care dollars being spent on? According to CIHI, most spending on health care continues to be for hospitals, drugs, and physician services. Over the last couple of years, the pace of spending on pharmaceuticals has increased and drugs are forecast to have the fastest growth rate of any of these three categories in the years to come.

CIHI's projections for the year 2017 — the last data available — looked like this:

- Hospital spending: 28.3 percent of total health expenditures; $1,871 per person; 1.9 percent annual growth per person.
- Drug spending: 16.4 percent of total health expenditures; $1,086 per person; 4.2 percent annual growth per person.
- Physician spending: 15.4 percent of total health expenditures; $1,014 per person; 3.4 percent annual growth per person.

But perhaps the two most alarming statistics that can be found on CIHI's website are the following:

- Total spending on health care in Canada is projected to reach $242 billion in 2017, with growth of around 3.9 percent. This will represent 11.5 percent of Canada's gross domestic product and equal $6,604 per Canadian.

- Spending on health care has trended upward since 1975, both in current dollars and in 1997 constant dollars. In current dollars, spending on health care reached $100 billion around 2000 and $200 billion around 2011.

Did you catch that? Let me repeat it for you, then. In current dollars, spending on health care reached $100 billion around 2000 and $200 billion around 2011. A $100 billion jump in just eleven years? And people think that's sustainable?

These aren't my numbers, by the way. I'm not making this stuff up. Again, the Canadian Institute for Health Information is one of the most trusted and respected health information/data metrics organizations in the world. If its numbers show Canada's health care system, as currently configured, is unsustainable, who am I to argue? And yet, there are those — some with an even bigger public profile than me, people like Dr. Danielle Martin and the Canadian Doctors for Medicare group, to name but two — who would have you believe the status quo is just fine, move along, people, there's nothing to be seen here.

Well, I'm sorry, but that's just not true. Unlike many of the so-called defenders of medicare, I actually run a business. I'm not feeding at the trough, picking money from the public purse, like that bunch. And as a person who runs a business, I know the importance of cash flow, stability, and sustainability when it comes to making plans for the future. I don't know how else to say it, but if the amount of money Canada is spending on health care doubled in eleven years, then there's no way in hell we're going to avoid that scary demographic iceberg waiting out there in the harbour, looking to sink us and everything we hold dear. And it's only going to get worse. So long as our leaders continue to turn a blind eye and pretend everything's A-OK, then I can guarantee you the whole thing's going to go down in flames by 2030 at the latest.

While you're digesting all that, here are some other numbers Dr. Brian Day shared with me that you might wish to consider:

- Private clinics in British Columbia perform more than sixty thousand operations a year, which saves the B.C. government more than $300 million annually.

- Of the 196 or so countries in the world, Canada is the only one that outlaws private insurance or personal spending on necessary health care.
- Seventy-six percent of Canadians think they should be able to buy private insurance for treatments outside the public system.
- Studies done in British Columbia show that public administration costs for health care are 15 percent, which is roughly double that of Medicare in the United States.
- Twenty-six percent of Canadian doctors have had a patient die on a wait-list.
- Canada has one health care civil servant for every 1,400 citizens, eleven times as many as in Germany, which has a hybrid system, universal care, and no wait-lists.

Pass the Alka-Seltzer, please.

The "Third Rail"

It's been said that health care is the "third rail" of Canadian politics. Dare to touch it and you'll wind up dead — especially if you're a politician. The phrase, most commonly attributed to the former speaker of the United States House of Representatives, Tip O'Neill, during the Ronald Reagan presidency, was actually coined in 1982 by O'Neill's aide — a fellow named Kirk O'Donnell — in reference to social security. O'Donnell was, of course, alluding to what happens when someone touches the high-voltage third rail, which provides the power to run most electric train systems in North America.

In Canada, the third rail metaphor has most often been used — rather effectively, I might add — to discourage anyone from suggesting our health care system, as it currently stands, is unsustainable; that the status quo is no longer an option; and that Canada is desperately in need of the hybrid solution. In fact, every time I suggest embracing the concept of a parallel private system to operate alongside our public one, my political friends typically turn a brighter shade of pale and start waving their arms like a person who can't swim and is about to go under for the third time. "No, no, no," they exclaim, "it'll never fly! The public won't accept it. We'd get killed at the polls." This, even though not a single one of them disagrees with me in private that a hybrid health care system is the way to go.

But if you stop for a moment and think about it, you'll come to realize that far from being a negative thing, touching the third rail can be a positive. While it's true that if a person or animal touches the third rail of a subway or other commuter train that runs on electricity at the same time they're touching one of the two rails the train travels on, they will be electrocuted, the fact is the third rail provides the power so the train can move forward. Or to put it another way, instead of thinking of the third rail as something *not* to be touched, we should instead start thinking of it as something that *must* be touched in order for the system to work at peak capacity.

One of the reasons wait-lists for surgery are so long in this country is that our provincial and territorial governments aren't able to provide adequate funds to hospitals to keep their operating rooms open and functioning more than one or two days a week. Imagine a system where some of the best surgeons in the world are not allowed to practise simply because the government can't find enough nickels and dimes to keep the lights on. Best health care system in the world? I hardly think so.

Of course, there are other problems besides inadequate funding; there's also the infrastructure deficit. Guess who pays for all those hospitals our elected officials are so proud of? We do. Not through taxes, though. Bricks and mortar are not funded by the government. Hospitals must put together foundations and recruit local civic leaders to help them endlessly badger citizens and businesses so they can raise the funds necessary to build a new hospital or add a wing to an old one. Oh sure, politicians will show up for the ribbon cutting once the facility is built and about to open — but will they actually cover the cost of the construction? Uh-uh.

While we're on the topic of paying for things, next time you visit your family doctor, take a look around and ask yourself one simple question: "Who's paying for all this?" The building, the office, the reception area, the waiting room, the equipment and technology, the cotton swabs and stethoscopes. You might think all these things would be covered by the government. But you would be wrong. Doctors provide billions — that's right, I said *billions* — of dollars of free infrastructure just so we, their patients, will have somewhere to go to access the health care system. And remember, we're just talking bricks and mortar here. I'm not even including the costs of paying for electricity, phones and fax machines, the internet, and salaries and benefits for their staff.

Instead of being grateful for all this, and offering up their sincere thanks, politician after politician will instead take every opportunity to vilify Canada's doctors, suggesting they don't care about their patients, they care only about money. Take Dr. Eric Hoskins in Ontario, for example. When he couldn't reach a deal at the negotiating table with the province's thirty thousand or so doctors, he called a media conference and shared billing information with the media on some of Ontario's top billers, claiming they were ripping off the system and pocketing millions of dollars a year. Dr. Hoskins implied that the average "salary" of an Ontario doctor was $368,000 per annum — leaving out the important detail that far from being a salary, that number represented the average amount *billed* by the average doctor yearly, before paying taxes and covering office salaries and overhead. Because the aforementioned expenses eat up anywhere between 40 and 60 percent of the amount of money billed by doctors, this means they'd have something closer to $150,000 to $200,000 at the end of the day — not $368,000. Oh, and by the way, no benefits, no pension, and no vacation pay, to boot.

But I digress.

The important thing — the point I'm trying to make here — is that the status quo is not working; it's not able to provide the care that people want and need. Dumping endless amounts of money into the system — if that were possible — would help a little, but obviously that's not an option. What's needed, to improve care and to reduce costs, is a radical rethink of how the system operates. Other options must be explored, because if we insist on sticking with the system we have, a system without choice, without freedom, and without flexibility, creativity, and innovation, we're doomed. Henry Ford was reported to have said, "If I had asked people what they wanted, they would have said faster horses." A funny line, to be sure. Unfortunately, this is the mindset of our elected officials and civil servants. They can't imagine any other way for the system to operate. But if real, positive change is to occur, we should embrace it with all our hearts and do so soon. Because the only way we're going to save medicare from itself and all those well-meaning but dangerous do-gooders is by performing some rather serious and radical surgery on it — *now* — before it's too late.

One thing that would help, needless to say, is if those who are in favour of propping up our current public health care system at all costs turned down the rhetoric just a tad. People like Dr. Brian Day and I are not unpatriotic, money-grubbing capitalists, who are looking to get rich on the backs of the sick and the poor. Far from it. The reality is our current system puts the vulnerable and disadvantaged in our society in a much worse place than if we actually had a hybrid system. After all, no one is suggesting for a minute that Canada adopt the broken and dysfunctional health care system of our neighbours to the south. No, what we're proposing here is to create something new and better — a made-in-Canada solution that takes the best ideas of other health care systems from around the world and combines them with Canadian values. That's the kind of health care system I'm talking about. Not a U.S.-style, two-tier one where people are judged by the size of their bank account instead their health care needs. If we don't wake up soon, however, we're going to find ourselves stuck with just that. It doesn't have to be that way. But I guarantee you it will be, if the defenders of medicare don't start listening a little more and talking a little less.

Who are these defenders? Dr. Danielle Martin is one.

I dubbed Dr. Martin "Medicare's Joan of Arc" in an article I wrote a few years back. There was quite an outcry at the time — especially from her supporters — mainly because I had the audacity to suggest that the good doctor would be wise to remember what happened to the original Joan of Arc. Those who fashion themselves defenders of Dr. Martin, and who apparently never learned about allegory or metaphor, took the line literally and were outraged that I seemed to be implying that medicare's number one advocate in Canada should be burned at the stake. I was, of course, suggesting no such thing. I was merely reacting to a speech Dr. Martin had given to Unifor's Ontario Regional Council in Port Elgin, Ontario: "In my view, it's the biggest threat to medicare in this generation," Dr. Martin told the more than six hundred Unifor members in attendance, referring to Dr. Brian Day's Charter challenge, "and we need to do everything we can to protect our health care system from the damage that its outcome could set in motion. This is not just a British Columbia issue. The ramifications will be felt across our entire country. If the case goes to the Supreme Court of Canada, there's the threat that the Canada Health Act itself may come under attack."

Unifor is Canada's largest private-sector union, with more than three hundred thousand members. Dr. Martin had been hoping for a $25,000 donation from the union to help defer her legal costs for defending the indefensible. Unifor committed to donating $50,000.

Shawn Rouse, Unifor's Ontario Health Care Council chair, described the threat of private clinics as "death by a thousand cuts" and warned that if the B.C. challenge was successful, privatization would inevitably cause a great deal of harm to our universal Canadian health care system. Darlene Prouse, Unifor Local 2458's second vice-president, also chimed in. "It must be our wake-up call that we could lose something that is dear to all of us," she said, urging her colleagues to join the fight. Dr. Martin concluded her remarks by telling the audience that Canada's universal, single-payer health care system is a reflection of our values as Canadians.

Oh, really? Come now, Dr. Martin. An insurance scheme is a reflection of our values as Canadians? Good God.

Look, I have nothing personal against Dr. Martin. She's a fine person — and a great talent — and I have no doubt she'll run for public office someday. In fact, I wouldn't be at all surprised to see her end up as a federal or provincial health minister somewhere down the road. But this madness has to stop. All the Canada Health Act does — if we're to be honest about it — is legislate equal access to what is fast becoming one of the worst health care systems in the world. I find it especially appalling that nowhere among the five principles of medicare — public administration, comprehensiveness, universality, portability, and accessibility — is there any mention of the word "quality." Which means, my friends, that when we're talking about Canada's health care system, someone who dies on a wait-list is no different from a patient with a successful outcome. Either way, everyone gets to move up a spot.

Are those Canadian values? It's certainly not Canadian common sense.

An Insurance Scheme, Not a System

When you go in search of a dictionary definition of the word "system," you'll find

- a regularly interacting or interdependent group of items forming a unified whole;

- an organized set of doctrines, ideas, or principles usually intended to explain the arrangement or working of a systematic whole;
- an organized or established procedure;
- harmonious arrangement or pattern; and
- an organized society or social situation regarded as stultifying or oppressive.

Of the five possibilities the dictionary offers up, it's the last definition — "an organized society or social situation regarded as stultifying or oppressive" — that comes the closest to describing the health care system we currently have in our country. Now, I probably don't have to spell this out for you but they're undoubtedly alluding to a political system like they had in Soviet Russia, or like they have today in China, or Cuba — in other words, *communism*.

Now, if one looks for a workable definition of the term "health care system," here's what the World Health Organization has to offer:

> A good health system delivers quality services to all people, when and where they need them. The exact configuration of services varies from country to country, but in all cases requires a robust financing mechanism; a well-trained and adequately paid workforce; reliable information on which to base decisions and policies; well maintained facilities and logistics to deliver quality medicines and technologies.

Sadly, this doesn't quite sound like what we have here in Canada.

There's a reason for that. Take a look at the Government of Canada's own website, where you'll find the following definition for the medicare system in Canada:

> Medicare is a term that refers to Canada's publicly funded health care system. Instead of having a single national plan, we have 13 provincial and territorial health care insurance plans. Under this system, all Canadian residents

have reasonable access to medically necessary hospital and physician services without paying out-of-pocket.

Roles and responsibilities for health care services are shared between provincial and territorial governments and the federal government.

The provincial and territorial governments are responsible for the management, organization and delivery of health care services for their residents.

The federal government is responsible for

- setting and administering national standards for the health care system through the Canada Health Act;
- providing funding support for provincial and territorial health care services;
- supporting the delivery for health care services to specific groups; and
- providing other health-related functions.

So, there you have it — straight from the horse's mouth, as it were. In Canada, we don't have a health care system. We have an insurance scheme, and — as I've said elsewhere — a badly run one, at that. Don't believe me? Read that second sentence over again. "Instead of having a single national plan, we have thirteen provincial and territorial health care insurance plans." It's like playing a hockey game with thirteen different sets of rules. In Toronto and Montreal, for instance, the game will be divided into three twenty-minute periods. But in Ottawa, Winnipeg, and Vancouver, fans will instead be forced to sit through four fifteen-minute quarters. While in Edmonton and Calgary, there will be no breaks at all — the game will simply go on until the full sixty minutes expire and a whistle blows, signalling the end of the match. Needless to say, no hockey fan would put up with this kind of craziness. And yet, this is exactly how our so-called health care "system" operates every day in Canada.

Otto von Bismarck, who was first chancellor of the German Empire from 1871 to 1890, once said, "Politics is the art of the possible." What he meant by this is quite simple. In politics, it doesn't matter what's right or what's wrong. The only thing that matters is results. Unfortunately, the problem with this approach, as I'm sure you'll agree, is that it ultimately leads to a series of compromises — and compromises, while they might be useful in helping build consensus, typically weaken the final product. As a former Canadian member of Parliament once explained to me, developing policy is a lot like decorating a Christmas tree. You start out with a tall and sturdy tree, one that stands upright and is noble and beautiful. But by the time everyone has had their say and decorated the tree in their own special way, that once beautiful Christmas tree is now bent over, the branches bending and almost breaking, the whole tree ready to collapse under the weight of so many contradictory and conflicting expectations.

If you think this sounds like a description of Canada's health care system, you're right. Because our leaders have had no backbone over the past fifty, sixty, seventy years, we've ended up with a system that isn't a system, a plan that appears to care more about tactics than actual strategy. This is hardly surprising. In my line of work, I see this all the time. Clients focus on details, without considering the bigger picture, and almost always mix up tactics and strategy. To put it in its simplest terms, a strategy is the plan you develop to accomplish something. The plan should contain specific goals, deliverables, and measurables, along with a timeline and a budget. Tactics, on the other hand, are the things you do to put your plan into action. These might include lobbying elected officials, holding a media conference, writing op-eds, or organizing rallies in front of provincial legislatures or on Parliament Hill in Ottawa. When you fall in love with tactics — which is quite easy to do and understandable, as I remind my clients most every day — you're likely to find yourself becoming more and more distracted and will inevitably take your eye off the ball.

This is what I suspect happened to medicare in Canada.

Our government has continually thrown good money after bad at our health care system. It didn't work then and it isn't working now. Unless we have the courage *and* integrity to admit our health care system *isn't* a system, that what we're doing *isn't* working, and are willing to tear it down and start all over again, then I'm afraid medicare as we know it is going to die a slow and painful death. We need to reinvent Canada's health care system. Simply tinkering at the edges, trying a tweak here and a tweak there, and making grandiose announcements just won't cut it. We need to be bold. We need to be brave. We need to, as I just said, not lose our focus but instead dig deeper until we unearth the *real* problem. Only then, by identifying where things have gone off the rails and exploring how we might truly reinvent Canada's health care system, will we be able to build a system that actually works. One we can all be proud of.

Nutrition, Wellness, and Prevention: The Flip Side of Sickness

To be perfectly honest, I'm probably the last guy you should be taking advice from when it comes to nutrition, wellness, and prevention. After all, I figure I've been committing suicide with food for most of the past fifty years or so. I eat too much red meat, consume too much sugar, and don't eat nearly enough fruit, vegetables, and grains. I love desserts. Cakes, cookies, brownies, tarts … you name it. And don't even get me started on cheese and chocolate. I'm such a foodaholic, I'll even *combine* cheese and chocolate, consuming both like some depraved king stuffing himself with all the treasurers of the hunt.

As for prevention and wellness, well … I think I can say with some degree of confidence that I never gave either much thought when I was growing up. Sure, my mother might have made me take some vitamin C in the wintertime, or perhaps a multivitamin if I was feeling sluggish and looking a little rundown but, for the most part, I mainly just tried not to hurt myself or get sick in the first place. Did it work? Sometimes, yes. And sometimes, no. I was often sick as a child — with the flu, mumps, measles, chicken pox … pretty much all the standard childhood diseases — and missed a lot of school. But I survived, like most every other member of my generation did. And I carried on for years, ignoring the inevitable and laughing in the face of fate. It didn't matter that my diet was atrocious or that there was a worrisome history of heart disease and stroke in my family. I walked five miles a day, and worked hard, and had energy to burn. Nothing was going to bring *me* down.

And then I turned forty. Almost as if someone had flipped a switch, the wheels started to come off and all those years of bad eating and abuse suddenly caught up with me. Kidney stones. High blood pressure. Knee, ankle, and foot problems. A hernia. Small things, by themselves. But cumulatively, each started to take a toll on me. I was in pain, so the doctors gave me painkillers. My blood pressure was so high, I could have "stroked out" at any moment. My lower-body problems were making it difficult to walk even one mile a day. I gained ten pounds, twenty pounds, thirty. Suddenly, eating a donut and a bag of Cheezies for breakfast wasn't so funny anymore. I had to stop equating food with love and contentment … because, frankly, food was no longer making me feel loved and content. It was killing me.

While the possibility of death was constantly on my mind during this time, pain was becoming a much bigger problem. When I had my first encounter with kidney stones, shortly after I turned forty, I was confused initially. I had cooked myself hamburgers for supper, then gone out for a walk, getting drenched by a surprise late-winter storm of freezing rain. I came home, had a hot shower, and went to bed. Then, shortly after eleven, I began to feel the symptoms. At first, I thought I'd caught a bug while sloshing my way through the storm. Then it occurred to me this might be what food poisoning feels like. I made my way to the bathroom, in hopes that throwing up might make me feel better. But I was in so much pain, I could neither kneel down nor stand up.

I decided I'd better make my way to the hospital, which, fortunately, was only a couple of blocks away, before I expired and someone found my body a few days later. It took me about fifteen minutes to cover the two blocks, shuffling my feet like the old man I wasn't but would one day become. I pretty much crawled into the hospital's emergency department, slapped my health card on the desk, and said, "I think I have food poisoning." They put me on a gurney and wheeled me into a room. About half an hour later, a doctor came in, took one look at me, and said, much to my surprise, "You're having a kidney stone attack."

"Kidney stones?" I replied. "But that's impossible." Turns out it wasn't.

I tell this story not because my situation is unique, but because it isn't. We are eating ourselves to death, getting next to no exercise, and doing the wrong things so often it's a wonder more of us aren't dropping like flies on a daily basis. If we're ever going to fix our health care system, we must first fix ourselves. In other words, we have to stop relying on others to keep us healthy. Remember, we don't have a health system. We have a *sickness* system. Doctors have neither the time nor financial incentive to keep us healthy. That's up to us. And just in case you think you can ignore what your body is trying to tell you, let me make this as clear as I can. I'm the poster boy for how not to live your life — at least when we're talking about nutrition, wellness, and prevention.

While it's true I never smoked, or abused drugs or alcohol (any more than the normal, socially awkward teenager might do growing up), the fact is a lack of physical activity and a lifetime of unhealthy eating made me a prime candidate to end up a perpetual patient. Today, at age sixty, my calendar is jam-packed with doctor appointments. Blood pressure monitoring and prescription renewals with my family doctor. Heart tests and follow-up consultations with my heart specialist. Ultrasounds, blood tests, and urine samples so my kidney specialist can keep a close eye on what's going on. And thousands of dollars of pills, powders, and potions. This is no way to live your life, trust me. And if I had it all to do over again, knowing what I know now, I'd have made some changes. No, not *some* changes. A lot of changes. Committing suicide with food? Hell, I wasn't just committing suicide. I might as well have been a serial killer or a mass murderer. Because the reality is you're not just killing yourself when you abuse your body and mind as I've done, you're also driving a stake right through the hearts of your loved ones.

Think I'm being a little overdramatic? Listen to this:

When I was in the ambulance being rushed to the hospital after suffering my V-tach attack, my better half was making her way in a cab to the emergency department with our boy, after having pulled him out of school. I didn't know this at the time — not until she divulged it to me months later — but she told Junior in the cab that she should have married me. What she was really saying, of course, was that she should have married me *before I died*. Think about that for a moment. Kind of brings a tear to the eye and puts a lump in your throat, doesn't it? Fortunately, I didn't die — *that* time — and we did get married a couple of years later. But things could just have easily turned out differently. Something my wife and I both recognize. This is why I'm taking better care of myself, in the hopes that I'll be around to celebrate many more wedding anniversaries and perhaps even the birth of our first grandchild someday.

Finding a Family Doctor and Dealing with Wait-Lists

Believe it or not, there was a time when Canada didn't suffer from a shortage of family doctors. In the early 1970s, Canadians enjoyed one of the highest physician-to-patient ratios in the developed world. Unfortunately, in the mid-1980s — around the time the Trudeau government introduced the

Canada Health Act and David Peterson took over as premier in Ontario — a few influential academics began to voice concern about what they considered to be Canada's oversupply of physicians — in particular, family doctors. As a result, Morris L. Barer and Greg L. Stoddart were commissioned by Canada's health ministries to produce a report that would examine the perceived problem and make recommendations. The two researchers delivered their report — a discussion paper that became known as the "Barer-Stoddart Report" — to a group of federal, provincial, and territorial deputy ministers of health in 1991.

The report recommended, among other things, slashing medical school enrolment by 10 percent, reducing the number of provincially funded post-graduate training positions by 10 percent, and reducing Canada's reliance on foreign-trained physicians. Not surprisingly, particularly in light of the fact that in the early 1990s Canada was in the throes of the worst economic downturn since the Great Depression, governments of all political stripes at both the provincial and federal levels of government were quick to act on Barer and Stoddart's recommendations, accepting all three of these recommendations, with the goal of maintaining or reducing the current physician-to-patient ratio in our country. Prior to making these changes, Canada's physician-to-patient ratio had continued to increase from the early 1960s to the late 1980s, peaking in 1993 at 2.1 physicians per 1,000 people. Since 1993, however, physician supply has been growing just fast enough to maintain a ratio of 2.1 physicians per 1,000 people.

So, it worked. Right? Wrong.

As a result of this short-sighted decision, Canada now has one of the lowest physician-to-patient ratios among nations that guarantee their citizens access to health care services regardless of ability to pay. Or, to put it another way, the policies that government embraced nearly thirty years ago have artificially restricted the growth rate of the physician-to-patient ratio in order to maintain a level that is below what other nations provide through their government-funded universal health care programs, resulting in a ratio that is significantly below the current demand for physician services in Canada. This, in a nutshell, is why so many Canadians continue to have a hard time finding a family doctor — despite the fact that many of those in charge of our health care system here in Canada have realized the error of their ways and have spent the last few years trying to minimize the damage caused by the mistake their predecessors made in the early 1990s.

The numbers from Statistics Canada, sadly, tell the story rather well:

- A total of 4.4 million Canadians, or 15 percent of the population aged twelve and older, report that they do not have a regular family doctor.
- Just over half (53 percent) of them say they have tried to find one. Among that group, 40 percent report that doctors where they live were not taking on new patients, 31 percent say their doctor had retired or left the area, while 27 percent claim there were no doctors available in their area.
- Of all the Canadians without a doctor, more than eight in ten say they have a place they usually go when they need medical care or health advice. Most (62 percent) identify that place as a walk-in clinic, while 13 percent say they go to a hospital emergency department when they are sick.
- Only 31 to 46 percent of Canadians, depending upon which province they live in, report being able to get an appointment to see their family doctor either the same day or the next day.
- Accessing medical care after hours without resorting to paying a visit to a hospital emergency department is difficult for 62 percent of Canadians.
- Almost half (49 percent) of Canadians aged fifty and over have never been screened for bowel or colon cancer.

Sobering numbers, indeed.

But finding a family doctor doesn't guarantee you timely access to treatment. No, no, no. This is Canada, and the harsh reality is, should your family doctor decide to send you to a specialist, you're going to learn what it means to wait. And wait. And wait. Never mind how much pain you're in. Never mind how much inconvenience and suffering your condition is causing you and your loved ones. In Canada, we ration health care in much the same way England and other countries rationed food during the Second World War and Soviet Russia rationed just about everything when the communists were running the show.

In a 2016 survey, the Fraser Institute found that here in Canada there was a median wait of twenty weeks — that's almost five months, folks — for "medically necessary" treatments and procedures. What makes this survey particularly useful is that it calculated total wait times faced by patients, starting from the time they received a referral from their family doctor, to their consultation with a specialist, to when they ultimately received treatment or underwent a procedure. Twenty weeks represents the longest-recorded wait time since the Fraser Institute first began tracking the issue in Canada and more than double the wait times reported in 1993. In a media release accompanying the survey, the Fraser Institute estimated that Canadians are currently waiting for nearly one million medically necessary procedures. To put this in perspective, most physicians will tell you that when patients are forced to wait three weeks or longer after seeing a specialist to be treated or have an operation their lives are potentially being put at risk because of unreasonable wait times. Again, the numbers paint a disturbing picture:

MEDIAN WAIT TIMES BY PROVINCE		MEDIAN WAIT TIMES BY SPECIALTY	
New Brunswick	38.8 weeks	Neurosurgery	46.9 weeks
Nova Scotia	34.8 weeks	Orthopaedic Surgery	38.0 weeks
P.E.I.	31.4 weeks	Ophthalmology	28.5 weeks
Newfoundland and Labrador	26.0 weeks	Plastic Surgery	25.9 weeks
		Otolaryngology	22.7 weeks
British Columbia	25.2 weeks	Gynecology	18.8 weeks
Alberta	22.9 weeks	Urology	16.2 weeks
Manitoba	20.6 weeks	Internal Medicine	12.9 weeks
Quebec	18.9 weeks	General Surgery	12.1 weeks
Saskatchewan	16.6 weeks	Cardiovascular	8.4 weeks
Ontario	15.6 weeks	Radiation Oncology	4.1 weeks
		Medical Oncology	3.7 weeks

Michael Decter, board chair of the advocacy group Patients Canada, responding to the Fraser Institute's survey results, said simply pouring more money into our health care system won't fix wait times. The proof, he said, is that despite the fact the federal government has increased health transfers to provinces by 6 percent a year for the past decade, wait times have gotten worse. "It's about innovation, it's about accountability, it's about focus and it's about transparency," he said. "It's not about more money." Decter then suggested that if governments were serious about fixing the problem, they'd offer patients something he calls "a safety guarantee." Any patient unable to access medically necessary treatment in a timely fashion would be transported to another province — or even another country — where wait times were more in line with what's considered acceptable.

Dr. Brian Day agrees that the problem isn't a lack of funding. "Studies show that Canada is one of the biggest spenders," he said, "but way down at the bottom when it comes to access and quality." The real problem, according to Dr. Day, is that governments in Canada have an iron-fisted monopoly on insuring health care, which can only lead to rationing of services and a lack of accountability.

Eyes and Teeth versus Pharmacare

Of all the developed countries in the world that have a universal health care system, Canada is the only one that doesn't cover prescription drugs. To make matters worse, Canadians pay some of the highest prices for those drugs in the world. Because of the way medicare was originally set up in this country, Canadians — no matter where they reside — are forced to navigate their way through a patchwork of public and private drug coverage programs, which all too often leave many of us on the outside looking in. According to one study, a quarter of Canadians who aren't covered by workplace insurance plans can't afford to fill their prescriptions, while 10 percent of those with insurance *still* find it difficult to pay for their drugs. Adding to the confusion, drugs that are covered by the government can vary from province to province.

Clearly, Canada needs a national pharmacare program. Or do we? It might surprise you that, given how many prescriptions I have to fill every month for myself and my family, I'm *not* in favour of going down that road. Even though I run my own small business and don't have enough employees to make it worth my while to pay for any sort of drug benefit plan, which means I have to pay for all this out of my own pocket, I can't justify bankrupting the country simply because my doctors have decided to turn me into a pill-popper.

Those in favour of introducing a national pharmacare program in Canada typically offer up the following four reasons for doing so: access to essential medicines is a human right; a national pharmacare program would save lives; implementation of such a program would save billions of dollars a year; and it would help Canadian businesses.

Let's take a closer look at each of these four arguments.

The World Health Organization (WHO) has decreed that access to essential medicines is a human right, and therefore recommends every country should introduce legislation that protects their citizens against the high cost of being uninsured, and develop pharmaceutical policies that go hand in hand with whatever other kinds of universal health care coverage a particular country offers its citizens.

As for the argument that having a national pharmacare program would help save lives, there could well be some truth to this, as studies have shown that Canadians are three to five times more likely to skip filling their prescriptions because of cost than those residing in countries offering universal coverage. A 2012 study showed that unequal coverage for adult Ontarians with diabetes was a contributing factor in the deaths of five thousand people between 2002 and 2008.

Not only would a universal pharmacare program save lives, it would also save Canadians huge amounts of money. Studies show that Canadians spend 50 percent more per capita on pharmaceuticals than those living in New Zealand, Sweden, and the United Kingdom, as well as a number of other countries with universal pharmacare programs. Or, to put it another way, we Canadians are spending an extra $12 billion a year simply because we don't have pharmacare.

The lack of a proper pharmacare system also costs Canadian businesses significant amounts of money. Currently, Canadian companies waste between $3 and $5 billion per year, mainly because the private insurance plans they've set up for their employees are unable to manage pharmaceutical costs effectively. When you factor in the alarming news that the number of prescription drugs costing more than $10,000 per year have grown almost tenfold in the past decade, it doesn't take a genius to figure out the effect this is having on the bottom line.

Good, solid arguments, one and all. And yet, I can't help thinking that there is a better way.

Before I share my solution to our national pharmaceutical nightmare with you, however, we really need to talk about two other rather important things … eyes and teeth.

To understand the lunacy of living in a country with a health care system that isn't really a system, one need look no further than the infuriating case of Balin Vergunst, a teenage boy who suffered from the progressive eye disease known as *keratoconus*, which causes the normally round cornea to thin and bulge, creating serious vision problems. As the condition worsened, the young boy struggled more and more in school and had to give up sports.

Balin's parents were given the following options by the Ontario government: pay thousands of dollars out of pocket for the surgery that could save their son's sight, or wait until he was legally blind, at which point the province's public health care system could help him.

The boy saw several specialists, including a pediatric ophthalmologist who recommended trying a minimally invasive procedure called corneal collagen cross-linking (or CXL for short), which could be done right away. CXL is not a new procedure, by the way. It's been performed in other parts of Canada for years with excellent results. Unfortunately, there was a slight catch. If they wanted the surgery performed, Balin's parents would have to cough up $3,000 because CXL isn't covered by the Ontario Health Insurance Plan (OHIP). If they chose not to do this, then, as previously mentioned, the parents could wait until the boy became legally blind, which would make him eligible for a costlier and more complicated procedure — a corneal transplant — a procedure that OHIP actually *does* cover. Not surprisingly, the parents borrowed money from family members in order to pay for the CXL procedure, which was successfully performed at the Ottawa Eye Institute.

Now, I grant you, not everyone is going to find themselves in the position young Balin Vergunst did — battling a rare condition, as well as politicians and a bureaucracy ill-equipped to look after their own citizens. But this is what happens when you have an insurance scheme masquerading as a health care system.

Obviously, eyes are important. So are teeth. Every bit as important as pharmaceuticals. Roughly a sixth of Canadians don't visit their dentist — assuming they even have one — on a regular basis because they can't afford the cost or don't have dental insurance. In Ontario alone, it's estimated that between two and three million people have not seen a dentist in the past year — mainly because they can't afford it. And while Ontario does offer some public dental programs, only children from low-income families who are under eighteen years of age or children whose family is on social assistance can access them. No province in Canada offers any form of dental health program for low-income adults or seniors. Because of this lack of coverage for those who are most vulnerable — people making minimum wage or less; seniors and the institutionalized elderly; new Canadians and Indigenous people — those who fall into these categories not surprisingly have the highest rates of tooth decay, dental pain, and gum disease.

This is a serious issue, because diseases of the mouth can have a huge effect on one's general health and overall well-being. Study after study has shown there is a definite link between poor oral health and the severity of chronic conditions such as diabetes, cardiovascular diseases, and respiratory diseases. Gum disease, gingivitis, and missing teeth can also affect a person's sense of self-worth, as well as their ability to get a job. After all, it's hard to put your best foot forward in a job interview when you're in pain and are afraid to smile for fear of looking like a hillbilly.

So, what happens when someone is suffering dental pain but can't afford to go to a dentist? Many visit their family doctors instead — costing our health care system even more — in hopes of getting help, while others try to self-medicate or go to "black market" dentists who aren't qualified to provide dental care. Just how big a problem is this? In 2014 there were more than two hundred thousand visits to Ontario physicians for gum and teeth issues. This means that approximately every three minutes, somewhere in Ontario, someone went to a doctor's office in search of care for a dental problem. Regrettably, most physicians are neither trained nor equipped to deal with diseases of the mouth, so they are unable to provide the appropriate treatment. And because the Ontario Health Insurance Plan pays family doctors $33.70 for a fifteen-minute patient visit, Ontario's health care system chalked up an extra $7.5 million worth of unnecessary costs in that year alone — all without being able to solve the patients' problems.

Eyes and teeth versus pharmacare. It shouldn't have to come down to this — choosing among the three — but the reality is we need to make some tough choices here. I believe — and remember, I'm the guy shelling out big bucks for prescription drugs for myself and my family — the

Canadian government should order all of our country's provinces and territories to start funding eye care and dental care immediately. This would save us a lot of money down the road and dramatically improve the quality of life for so many of our fellow Canadians. As for introducing a national pharmacare program, we should be creative and do the following. One, educate Canadians on the high cost of drugs — especially those meant to combat preventable illnesses and conditions, like high blood pressure, smoking-related lung disease, and obesity. Two, make nutrition, wellness, and prevention a part of everyone's everyday life — instead of treating these things like an afterthought the way we do now. And three — and this is the big one — give Canadians the right to pay for their own health care by allowing them to open up medical savings accounts (MSAs), as part of a hybrid health care system, so that we can all take a bit more responsibility for the cost of our own dubious life decisions. (More on this later.)

A national pharmacare program? Not today, thanks. Although I have no problem with a program that would cover the costs of prescriptions for anyone over sixty-five years of age, or anyone making less than $30,000 a year. Covering eyes and teeth, on the other hand … well, to me that's a no-brainer. Hopefully, our elected officials and civil servants will figure it out before the bleeding-heart liberals and left-leaning socialists find yet another way to bankrupt the country they claim to love so much.

Dr. Google

We've all done it. Maybe your back is hurting. Or your new baby is suffering from diaper rash. Or you think you've got an ingrown toenail. Whatever the complaint, "Dr. Google" is available to offer up its diagnosis 24/7.

A year or two ago, I discovered, much to my chagrin, that I was starting to lose my words. So, being a modern man, I went to my computer, got on the internet and googled "losing my words." And there it was — primary progressive aphasia (or PPA, for short). "Primary progressive aphasia is a form of cognitive impairment that involves a progressive loss of language function," I read. "PPA begins very gradually and initially is experienced as difficulty thinking of common words while speaking or writing. It progressively worsens to the point where verbal communication by any means is very difficult." *Yikes*. Reading further, I discover that adults of any age can develop primary progressive aphasia, but that it's more common in people under the age of sixty-five. That's me.

I scrolled down the page and stopped when I came to a section called "Symptoms & Causes." Like most everyone else, I suspect, I placed a mental check mark beside the symptoms I thought I was exhibiting. Word-find hesitations. Check. Substitution of words (e.g., "table" instead of "chair"). Check. Using words that are mispronounced or incomprehensible (e.g., "track" for "truck"). Check. Talking around a word (e.g., "We went to the place where you can pick up food" for the words "grocery store"). Forgetting the names of familiar objects. Inability to think of names of people, even though the person is recognized. Check, check, check. Scrolling down further, I discovered that people with PPA tend to have similar clusters of symptoms. Researchers who specialize in PPA, it told me, currently recognize three subtypes: agrammatic, logopenic, and semantic. I didn't bother to stop and investigate any of these. Instead I carried on right to the bottom, looking for cures and treatments, only to discover there are none. Returning to the top of the page, I read that in many instances the person with PPA may be the first to note that something is wrong and the complaints may initially be attributed to stress or anxiety.

Aha, I thought. *There it is. Proof positive that I'm suffering from PPA.* Moments later, my wife came into the office and I broke the sad news that I had PPA.

"What is PPA?" she asked, reasonably enough.

"It's …" I replied, then stopped. "I forget what the individual letters stand for, but you can rest assured that I've got it."

My wife raised an eyebrow, and asked — again, quite reasonably — how I knew all this. "Have you been to the doctor?" she asked.

"No," I responded, "I read about it on Google."

She shook her head and told me I might want to get a second opinion, "like, from a real doctor, instead of just Dr. Google."

Not surprisingly, this use of the internet by the general public for self-diagnosis (or, more commonly, self-misdiagnosis) drives doctors crazy. Patients make an appointment for whatever's ailing them — real or imaginary — and then show up armed with pages and pages of information, most of it totally useless, demanding their doctor order some sort of test or prescribe some kind of pill so they can be cured of whatever it is as soon as possible. And while Dr. Google does, occasionally, make the right diagnosis, the treatment recommended might well leave something to be desired. Depending upon what medications a patient is already on — and rare is the person who isn't already taking something — adding a new pill might prove to be dangerous. Same with ordering tests. Most doctors will typically order up the least expensive test first in order to eliminate certain things and help preserve our precious health care dollars. Unfortunately, modern patients — especially those who've been to see Dr. Google beforehand — aren't interested in waiting around for results. They want answers now, damn the torpedoes.

Not every doctor is against this new, high-tech revolution, however.

Take Dr. Eric Topol, an American cardiologist and professor, for instance. In his book *The Patient Will See You Now*, Dr. Topol chided his fellow physicians for being so slow to embrace new technologies, giving as an example the time he received a text message from a patient that included a screenshot of an electrocardiogram he'd run on himself from a smartphone app. "I'm in Afib," the patient texted, referring to atrial fibrillation. "Now what do I do?" Dr. Topol clearly isn't one to mince words, proclaiming, "The digitisation of human beings will make a parody out of 'doctor knows best.' We're all essentially surgically connected to our smartphones and we're still in the early stages of realizing their medical potential."

Dr. Michael Gannon, former president of the Australian Medical Association, goes a step further, saying doctors should not be annoyed at patients who Google their symptoms before making an appointment. "What's difficult for patients is to work out what's a credible source of information and what's not." When asked if he uses the internet for his own research and to better understand unusual conditions, Dr. Gannon replied, "Look, I use Wikipedia frequently when I'm looking up rare genetic syndromes." The doctor went on to say that instead of being upset when someone walks in and says they've done their own research and decided they were "an expert," doctors should embrace the fact that people are trying to become more literate about their health.

Richard Worzel, who bills himself as Canada's leading futurist, thinks the sky's the limit when it comes to embracing technological advances in health care. By 2035, he predicts, there will be a global computer network that gathers information about the health of each individual within the network in order to provide early warning signs about possible new diseases or epidemics. This information will be shared with what Worzel calls "health-bots," national computer agents that search for patterns to determine if something is indeed a new disease, a mutation of an existing disease, or merely the seasonal re-emergence of a known disease. Still with me? National health-bots will then merge this information with global health-bots so that we humans can ultimately figure out what to do about it.

Pretty neat, huh?

It will also be possible to monitor our day-to-day health. Within ten to fifteen years, Worzel suggests, it'll only cost around $100 to decode someone's genome. As a result, normal, everyday people will have the ability to monitor their own heartbeats, see if they are having any fluctuations in body temperature, or are showing signs of any other abnormality. This detailed, individual monitoring of our health will lead to a noticeable reduction in things like heart attacks, strokes, and other "sudden onset" health threats like aneurysms, as well as identify early signs of any other forms of health troubles. Worzel even thinks that new breakthroughs in health care technologies will allow us to reprogram an individual's genetic code, so that cancer, diabetes, cystic fibrosis, multiple sclerosis, celiac disease, or other genetically linked diseases will be things of the past.

Taking it a step further, the futurist believes that eventually age will be treated in the same way we treat diseases. Organs, joints, and other body parts will be routinely replaced using new parts grown from a patient's own stem cells, which will have the obvious advantage of overcoming the problems of immune-system rejection we currently face. This means citizens will be able to live to be 120 and beyond — good news, but a development that will create its own set of problems, as Worzel is quick to point out. For example, if a person works and pays taxes from age twenty-five to sixty-five, as is the current reality for most of us, where is the money going to come from to pay them a pension for the next fifty-five years — especially when there's already a dearth of taxpaying workers coming along behind the baby boomers?

While all this might sound like an episode of *The X-Files* — in other words, the work of an overactive imagination — we'd be wise to keep in mind that to future generations our current advances in microsurgery, chemotherapy, and insulin monitoring may well seem as barbaric as the practice of bloodletting from previous centuries. I can't help remembering that scene from the fourth Star Trek movie, *The Voyage Home*, in which Captain Kirk and some crew members — including "Bones," the ship's doctor — return from the twenty-third century to 1986 San Francisco in order to save the Earth by enlisting the help of the only beings — humpback whales — who can communicate with an alien probe. Before the crew can successfully complete its mission, however, they must first save Chekov, who has been hurt in an accident, from the "barbarism" of twentieth-century medicine. Walking down the hospital corridor, searching for Chekov, Bones comes across a patient lying on a stretcher in the hallway and asks the woman what's wrong with her. "Kidney dialysis," she whispers. "Dialysis!" the doctor exclaims. "My God, what is this … the Dark Ages?" It's a scene played for laughs, to be sure. But in the brave new health care world of the future, what we're doing to one another today in the name of treating sickness and disease might not seem nearly so funny.

"Cancer Inc."

You're not going to like what I have to say. Not one bit. But the truth is it's time to put an end to the annual Terry Fox Run. The Terry Fox Run, for those who've spent the last thirty-plus years hiding in the jungle, is a non-competitive charity event that takes place in September each year all across Canada and in various countries around the world. The event commemorates a true Canadian hero, Terry Fox, and his incredible Marathon of Hope — a journey that began in St. John's, Newfoundland, in April of 1980, and ended in Thunder Bay, Ontario, in September of that same year. Fox, who'd lost his right leg to cancer, planned to run across Canada to raise funds for cancer research. Sadly, the cancer returned in September of 1980, forcing Terry to abandon his run — roughly at the halfway point — and seek treatment, after having covered 5,373 kilometres over 143 days. He died on June 28, 1981.

That might have been the end of the story had it not been for Isadore Sharp, founder of the Four Seasons Hotels. Sharp, who'd lost his own son to cancer, donated $10,000 and challenged 999 other businesses to do the same. He also proposed setting up an annual fundraising run in

Fox's name. Despite opposition from the Canadian Cancer Society and other charities, who feared the event would severely hamper their ability to raise funds for their own causes, the run went ahead on September 13, 1981, raising $3.5 million. Schools were encouraged to participate in the Terry Fox Run the following year. In the first six years alone, these National School Run Days raised over $20 million. By 1999, the Terry Fox Run had gone international, with over a million people in sixty countries participating. All in all, the Terry Fox Foundation has raised over $600 million for cancer research since the first Terry Fox Run. According to the organization's website, eighty-two cents of every dollar raised goes to cancer research, which is truly admirable. And as of 2017, nearly 1,300 separate cancer research projects have been funded by the foundation. In fact, in 2016 alone, the Terry Fox Foundation invested an estimated $26.6 million in three key areas of cancer research. These include discovery research, transitional research, and training future leaders.

So, what's my beef? Why do I feel this phenomenally successful Canadian institution should be put out to pasture?

It's simple, really. When it comes to finding a cure for cancer, we've failed. This is not to say that there haven't been some breakthroughs and significant discoveries as a result of all the money the Terry Fox Foundation has been pouring into cancer research over the past thirty-eight years. But let's face it. A "cure" is nowhere in sight. Now, while the conspiracy theorist in me would love to suggest somebody has already come up with a cure for cancer, and that the cure is being suppressed in order to ensure that the steady flow of all those millions of dollars being poured into cancer research doesn't suddenly dry up, alas, I don't believe it's true. No, I'm quite convinced that despite having some of our best people working on this problem, no one as of yet has come up with a cure for cancer, mainly because they haven't yet sufficiently nailed down what causes it.

So, while the Terry Fox Foundation has done an admirable job of keeping Terry's name and legacy alive over the past four decades, the time has come to retire the Terry Fox Run. If only because we're tired of being shaken down each year, guilted into paying a "Fear Tax." Which, if we're willing to be honest, is the real reason we donate to the Terry Fox Run. If we make a donation, the thinking goes, and pay the Fear Tax, we or one of our loved ones won't be struck down by cancer. Well, guess what? Having lost my father and brother to cancer and having watched my other brother and myself wage our own battles against skin cancer — all while giving generously to the Terry Fox Foundation over the years — I'm here to tell you that whether you pay now or pay later, cancer is still likely to catch up with you or someone you know and love eventually. It's inevitable. So, let's put an end to the fantasy that says there's a cure for cancer and it's right around the corner. And at the same time, let's have the decency to allow a great Canadian and true hero to finally rest in peace instead of rolling him out each September — like Lazarus risen from the dead — to shill for cancer research.

Terry deserves better than that. And so do we.

•••

The fact is, like the War on Drugs, the War on Cancer has proven to be a colossal failure. In the nearly six decades since former U.S. president Richard Nixon told the nation he'd be asking Congress for an extra $100 million to launch a campaign to find a cure for cancer, it's clear we're no closer to finding a cure today than when Nixon announced he was declaring, on behalf of all Americans, war on this most insidious and baffling of diseases. "The time has come in America," he told reporters, "when the same kind of concentrated effort that split the atom and took man to the moon should be turned toward conquering this dread disease."

Later that year — on December 23, 1971, to be precise — President Nixon, upon signing the National Cancer Act, told those gathered, "I hope in the years ahead we will look back on this action today as the most significant action taken during my administration."

For those who may not remember, the legislation gave the National Cancer Institute (NCI) special budgetary powers and allowed the NCI's director to report directly to the president. Not surprisingly, as seems to be the case with all wars, President Nixon's War on Cancer turned out to be something of a money pit. Today, the National Cancer Institute's annual budget is just north of $5 *billion* — and even that, according to those in the know, isn't nearly enough to carry on the fight. Now, I'm not looking to slag all those researchers who're working hard to find a cure. Nor do I wish to disparage the efforts of the many volunteers who continue to walk, run, and plead with the rest of us to pony up whatever we can spare in order to help feed the beast otherwise known as cancer research. But the fact is, if an investor was getting as poor a return on his or her investment as the general public is when it comes to cancer, he or she would've pulled the plug long ago.

So, let me be frank with you.

In 2019, I've come to the conclusion that instead of trying to find a cure for cancer — or worse, sitting on a cure without sharing it with the world because Big Pharma can't figure out how to monetize it — we should be investing time and money into *preventing* cancer. And while I understand some will think I've lost my mind here, suggesting that we stop looking for a cure and instead concentrate on ways we might prevent cancer, let me explain where I'm coming from. Having watched my brother fight a losing battle with metastatic melanoma for over a year; doctors giving him false hope as each new therapy was proposed, tried, and then ultimately abandoned; poisoning him with radiation and chemotherapy, before chopping out body parts as a last resort, I can't help thinking the cure was worse than what was ailing him.

• • •

Regrettably, not everyone believes "prevention is the new cure" when it comes to fighting cancer. Take the Ontario Liberal government, for instance. In 2015, they brought in the Making Healthier Choices Act, which, among other things, made it illegal to display or promote the use of e-cigarettes, and imposed age and other restrictions around their use. Many felt this bill was unconstitutional and wouldn't stand up to a court challenge, because it limits the rights of those wishing to replace regular cigarettes with e-cigarettes in hopes of reducing their chances of being diagnosed with lung cancer at a later date. At a time when the City of Toronto was considering a proposal from their chief medical officer of health, Dr. David McKeown, to allow three so-called safe injection sites to be set up in Toronto as a way of preventing deaths from overdoses and the spread of AIDS through the use of dirty needles, the Province of Ontario appeared to be heading in the opposite direction when it came to preventing lung cancer as a result of tobacco use. Each year, tobacco claims thirteen thousand lives in Ontario

— equivalent to thirty-six lives every day. Care to guess how many people die from drug overdoses in Ontario during a typical year? Most estimates peg it at somewhere between five hundred and six hundred per annum. So why, then, are our elected officials so determined to help drug addicts keep from killing themselves when they're putting so many unnecessary roadblocks in the way of those addicted to tobacco products, who I'm sure would like to keep from killing themselves, as well?

I have a theory.

There's no tax on illegal drugs. There *is*, however, tax on cigarettes — at least, on those sold over the counter and not on First Nations reserves. Could it be that the Government of Ontario has an addiction problem of its own? Might it not be just as addicted to the millions of dollars — if not *hundreds* of millions — of tax revenues that come into its coffers as a result of all those legal cigarettes being sold in the province? Makes you wonder, doesn't it? Because, frankly, the science the Ontario government has used to justify banning e-cigarettes is junk science at best. But according to a number of heralded studies conducted in the United Kingdom, electronic cigarettes, unlike real cigarettes, contain no carcinogens and there is zero evidence that exposure to second-hand vapour poses any health risks.

Thanks to our leaders' short-sightedness, I'm sorry to say, tens of thousands of Canadians are going to be felled by lung cancer unnecessarily — putting a huge financial strain on our already overburdened health care system — all because political meddling and bureaucratic game-playing has once again resulted in bad public policy and flawed legislation. It's enough to make you sick … but that's the way it is with the War on Cancer — and, indeed, all wars. Some people get rich. A bunch of people die. A bunch more are wounded. While the rest of us just stand around and shake our heads and wonder why. A never-ending cycle, I'm afraid, unless we someday find the courage to stand up and ask, "What are we fighting for?" Otherwise, we're going to come to regret ever taking part in this war — especially if we continue to blindly fill up the coffers of both government and that loathsome cottage industry known as "Cancer Inc."

Medical Assistance in Dying

There's a great short story by Kurt Vonnegut Jr. called "2 B R 0 2 B." Published in 1962, the story revolves around a man named Edward K. Wehling Jr., whose wife is about to give birth to triplets. In this bizarre world of the future, no child is allowed to survive unless his parents can find someone who'll voluntarily be put to death in order to make room for the new arrival. The title, which is a play on William Shakespeare's famous "To be or not to be" soliloquy from *Hamlet*, is also the phone number for the Federal Bureau of Termination (2 B or naught 2 B — get it?), where those who've decided they've had enough can call up and make an appointment to be euthanized. I won't spoil the tale for those of you who haven't read it by giving away the ending, but suffice to say that by the story's conclusion Vonnegut leaves us wondering if perhaps the best thing we can do for our loved ones is to hurry up and die — *now* — before it's too late.

•••

True, there are a lot of advantages to being the baby in the family. Folks will travel from all corners of the globe to bestow gifts upon you. There'll be lots of hugs and kisses from aunts and uncles and grandparents, and even from a whole bunch of people you don't know, and who you might never see again. And if you're lucky, like me, you'll have a couple of wonderful older brothers or sisters to show you the ropes, once you're old enough to walk and talk. In my case, I developed a lifelong love of sports thanks to my two brothers. I also learned what it means to be part of a loving family and why it's important to stick together — in good times and in bad.

Especially bad.

One of the not-so-good things about being the baby in the family is that, unfortunately, you end up having a number of people die on you over the years. All four of my grandparents have departed — my mom's dad having succumbed to his third and final stroke in October of the year I was born — as well as several aunts and uncles, both my parents, and one of my brothers. When it comes to death and dying, I've seen a thing or two.

As must be obvious by now, I'm the kind of guy who has an opinion on just about everything — and if I don't have an opinion on something, I'll come up with one right quick if you'll just give me a few minutes. In the case of euthanasia, I can't for the life of me understand what all the fuss is about. I mean, all you have to do is study a little history to see just how tied up in knots we've been about the whole right-to-die issue. For instance, in 1992, Sue Rodriguez, a woman living in British Columbia, asked the Supreme Court of Canada to allow someone to aid her in ending her life after she was diagnosed with ALS. Although the court refused her request in 1993, Ms. Rodriguez succeeded in ending her life a year later with the help of an unknown doctor. Shortly thereafter, Robert Latimer, a Saskatchewan farmer, was convicted of second-degree murder in the 1993 death of his daughter Tracy. The case sparked a national debate on the definition and ethics of euthanasia, as well as on the rights of the disabled.

Want more?

In 1996, Austin Bastable drove from his home in Windsor, Ontario, to Detroit, Michigan, where he died in the home of Janet Good with the assistance of Dr. Jack Kevorkian (a.k.a. Dr. Death). In 2006, seventy-seven-year-old John McCadden from Penticton, B.C., shot his eighty-year-old wife, Lorna, and then took his own life in a murder-suicide. Lorna had recently been diagnosed with Alzheimer's. In 2007, sixty-six-year-old Percy Stein, who lived in downtown Toronto, shot his eighty-four-year-old mother, Sarah, and then killed himself. He was in the final stages of advanced stomach cancer and his mother had suffered a stroke. Stein was his mother's primary caregiver, as he had never married.

Now, despite what many would have you believe, it wasn't against the law to kill yourself here in Canada — not since 1972, at any rate — before the Supreme Court of Canada forced the Government of Canada to act on the issue in 2015. Physician-assisted suicide, however, *was* illegal. According to the original version of Section 14 of Canada's Criminal Code (which has since been updated): "No person is entitled to consent to have death inflicted on him, and such consent does not affect the criminal responsibility of any person by whom death may be inflicted on the person by whom consent is given." Further, Section 241 (which has also now been updated) said: "Everyone who counsels a person to commit suicide or aids or abets a person to commit suicide, whether suicide ensues or not, is guilty of an indictable offence and liable to imprisonment for a term not exceeding fourteen years." All that changed, of course, on June 10, 2012, when the Supreme Court of British Columbia struck down those sections on constitutional grounds. Three years later, on February 6, 2015, the Supreme Court of Canada, in the case of *Carter v. Canada*, also struck down provisions prohibiting assisted suicide.

Arguments *for* euthanasia typically go something like this: Those who're in favour will make either the ethical argument or the pragmatic argument — or both. The ethical argument says everyone should have freedom of choice, including having control over their own body and life (so long as they're not violating the rights and freedoms of others) and that the government has no business creating laws that keep us from being able to choose how and when we die. Similarly, the pragmatic argument says since euthanasia (and particularly "passive" euthanasia, where medical treatment is deliberately withheld in order to hasten the patient's death) is already a fairly widespread practice throughout the world — albeit not one people are willing to acknowledge exists — we'd be wise to go ahead and regulate it in order to ensure those who're too sick to carry on can be dispatched to the next world safely and with dignity.

These arguments make a lot of sense to me. We *should* be able to choose the time, the location, and the method of our death — especially when the quality of our lives is in jeopardy. If fate deals one a bad hand and life is no longer worth living, why prolong the agony? Milan Kundera once said, "Dogs do not have many advantages over people, but one of them is extremely important: euthanasia is not forbidden by law in their case; animals have the right to a merciful death."

Those *against* euthanasia offer arguments that most often fall into the following four categories: the religious argument, the "slippery slope" argument, the medical ethics argument, and the "alternative" argument. According to the religious argument, human beings are created by God — and are, hence, sacred — and only God can decide when life should end. Therefore, those who commit an act of euthanasia, or otherwise assist in a suicide, are acting against the will of God and sinning. According to the slippery slope argument, once a government starts sanctioning the killing of its own citizens, a line is crossed that will ultimately set a dangerous precedent. To wit, someone in need of constant care, or suffering from a severe disability, might choose euthanasia so as not to be such a financial burden to their loved ones. The medical ethics argument claims that asking physicians to abandon their obligation to preserve life could put the doctor-patient relationship at risk. In other words, the physician might decide euthanasia is the best course of action simply as a way of saving the health care system money. Finally, the alternative argument declares that we shouldn't be so quick to overlook the value of palliative care when it comes to easing suffering for the sick and the dying, as it just might be a better option than euthanasia.

These arguments, to be perfectly honest, make little or no sense to me. While I respect the right of everyone to believe whatever they wish, I'm afraid that, as an atheist, I have to reject the concept we must continue to suffer needlessly because it's somehow "God's will." Similarly, I have a hard time understanding the "slippery slope" argument. I believe legalizing euthanasia actually goes a long way toward ensuring we *don't* put ourselves in a position where unscrupulous governments take advantage of the sick and the dying in order to balance the books. Just as legalizing abortion made it safer for women to get help without having to turn to "back-alley butchers," this too could be a good thing for society. As for the last two arguments against euthanasia, they're pretty much red herrings, as far as I can see. No one is asking physicians to do anything they don't feel comfortable with, nor is anyone downplaying the role those providing palliative care to our sickest and most vulnerable play, or suggesting there's no place for them.

But don't take my word for it.

Instead, I'd rather you listen to what the late infectious disease specialist Dr. Donald Low had to say about legalizing physician-assisted death, in a video he made just days before he succumbed to brain stem cancer on September 18, 2013. Dr. Low, as many of you will remember, became famous not just to Canadians but to the world at large, as a calming influence during the SARS crisis in Toronto in the winter of 2003. In his video, he said he would've liked to have the option of deciding when and how he was going to die and being able to enlist the help of another physician so he could fall asleep peacefully, surrounded by his family.

"In Canada, it's illegal," Dr. Low said, "and it'll be a long time before we mature to a level where we accept dying with dignity. I really envy countries like Switzerland and the Netherlands and the United States where this is possible. Why make people suffer for no reason when there's an alternative? I just don't understand it." Dr. Low continued, saying he hoped his death would be painless and perhaps would come in his sleep.

"I would hope that I'm able to face death without the fear of death itself. I'm not afraid of dying. I could make that decision tomorrow. I just don't want it to be a long, protracted process where I'm unable to carry out my bodily functions and talk with my family and enjoy the last few days of my life." He concluded his remarks by saying, "There's a lot of opposition to it. There's a lot of clinicians in opposition to dying with dignity. If they could live in my body for twenty-four hours, I think they would change that opinion."

Sums up rather nicely, don't you think, just how politicized the whole euthanasia debate had become before the federal government finally passed a bill on June 17, 2016, to legalize and regulate assisted dying. Unfortunately, the new legislation — as it currently stands — remains deeply flawed for a variety of reasons. In particular, despite recommendations from its own parliamentary committee, the government created legislation that doesn't permit mature minors, people suffering from mental illness, or those *not* currently suffering from a terminal illness but who are likely to be at a future date (when they'll be incapacitated and unable to make a clear-headed decision) the right to choose to die. If the government doesn't come to its senses someday soon and revisit the legislation — before the courts do it for them — ordinary Canadians like you and me who fall into the aforementioned categories will be forced to take measures into our own hands.

And in case you think I'm talking out of my hat, let me share my story.

I turned sixty years old on December 31, 2018. I've got a wonky heart, barely functioning kidneys, arthritis, skin cancer, and I come from a family with a history of stroke. To make matters worse, I'm nineteen years older than my wife, and thirty-eight years older than my stepson. And while I love life and continue to live it to the fullest, you don't need a crystal ball to figure out things are going to end badly for me. When that time finally comes, I hope my wife and stepson will be able to end my suffering legally, safely, and sanely, without having to worry about the ramifications or the possibility of facing criminal charges for engaging in what, when you stop and think about it, is the ultimate act of love. And for those of you who believe in God, and who say suicide — and especially *assisted* suicide — is a sin, let me ask you a question: What kind of God would allow people to suffer like that? To what end? For what purpose? It's time we acknowledged that death is as much a part of life as being born. Kill me softly … but kill me. Let me go out on my own terms, not those of some cowardly politician or imaginary man in the clouds.

We all deserve that much. At a minimum.

Three Health Care Tsunamis: Obesity, Diabetes, and Dementia

Three health care tsunamis — obesity, diabetes, and dementia — are waiting for us, for boomers and zoomers especially, looming just on the horizon, building up speed, and threatening to swamp our health care system and wipe out the treasury. These giant waves of trouble will be like nothing we've seen before or could possibly imagine. They will place incredible strains on the system, as health care professionals — doctors, nurses, physiotherapists, and personal support workers — try to deal with an overwhelming patient load, as well as a health care system ill-prepared to deal with these three disasters.

While some would argue that none of these problems exist — or at least, if they do exist, aren't nearly as bad as I'm suggesting — the evidence says otherwise. Today, one in four Canadian adults, for instance, and one in ten Canadian children, are considered to be clinically obese, according to the Canadian Obesity Network. So, upward of six million Canadians who've been diagnosed with obesity may need immediate assistance in dealing with their weight problems. The costs related to this alone — to mention nothing of the cost of other diseases and conditions associated with obesity, such as heart disease, stroke, arthritis, and cancer — are staggering. One report estimates that these costs account for $6 billion annually — that's 4 percent of the total Canada spends on health care. Even more alarming, this amount doesn't account for things like lost productivity, a reduction in tax revenues, or social costs.

My own "battle of the bulge" is quite instructive, and I suspect mirrors the experiences of many of my fellow Canadians. When I was a child, growing up in the 1960s, no one ever talked about nutrition, although I do recall seeing a chart somewhere in my classroom listing the four basic food groups: protein, such as meats, poultry, fish, dry beans and peas, eggs, and nuts; dairy products, such as milk, cheese, and yogurt; grains; and fruits and vegetables. I ate too much dairy and not enough fruits and veggies, snacked often, and had something of a pot-belly until I was twelve years old, when I miraculously grew almost a foot in one year, reaching my current height of six foot two by the time I hit high school. Regrettably, I didn't change my eating habits and so continued to put on weight. By the time I was in my mid to late twenties, I was having a hard time holding my weight under two hundred pounds. Finally, desperate to find something that might work, I went on a "cleansing" diet, losing forty pounds in one month, going from 210 to 170. Not surprisingly, once the diet was over, I yo-yoed back up to 210, then 220, then 230 — eventually topping out at 250 pounds. While I've managed to get rid of thirty of those unwanted pounds, it's been a constant battle and one filled with worry. For one thing, I'm concerned about the amount of damage all that extra weight is doing to my heart and joints. I'm especially concerned about having to deal with diabetes, what with the onset of old age. Several members of my family had or have it and I've been borderline diabetic for years.

Which brings us to the second health care tsunami we need to talk about. Between 1999 and 2009, the rate of diabetes among Canadians jumped 70 percent, according to the Canadian Diabetes Association (now Diabetes Canada). As a result of this astonishing growth, it's estimated that 2.4 million Canadians are now suffering from some form of diabetes — in other words, nearly 7 percent of the population. To put this in perspective, in the province of Ontario alone, the medical costs of dealing with those with diabetes are twice that of the general population. Mortality rates are also double those of the rest of us. Even worse, as revealed in a 2012 report by the auditor general of Ontario, people with diabetes are responsible for 69 percent of amputations, 53 percent of kidney dialysis, 39 percent of heart attacks, and 35 percent of strokes. But wait, there's more. Again, in Ontario, it's estimated that the number of people with diabetes will reach 1.9 million by the year 2020, up from 1.2 million in 2010 and 546,000 in 2000.

Those are astounding figures.

Sadly, diabetes, which is the result of one's inability to maintain normal blood-sugar levels, is something of a "silent" killer; it sneaks up on people, numbing nerves in the feet, damaging retinas, and screwing with the cardio-vascular system. Diabetes can also cut off circulation to our limbs, as well as wreak havoc on our kidneys. Even more troubling, it's estimated that in addition to those suffering with the disease now, more than five million Canadians — that's 15 percent of the country's population — are "prediabetic," and many of those are young adults and children. And yet, to most of us, diabetes is pretty much an unknown disease. Don't believe me? Remember the widespread panic during the swine flu outbreak a few years back? Fewer than five hundred Canadians died during the H1N1 flu pandemic from 2009 to 2010. During that same time period, approximately forty thousand Canadians died as a result of complications caused by diabetes. Even HIV/AIDS — as heartbreaking and devastating a disease as it's been over the years — isn't as big a threat in this day and age as diabetes is, although you wouldn't know it based on the coverage it gets in the media.

The third tsunami we must concern ourselves with is dementia. One study predicts that by the year 2050, 135 million people around the world will be living with dementia. In 2013, that number was forty-four million. By 2030, it's expected to jump to seventy-six million. This is frightening stuff, especially when you consider how woefully unprepared we are to deal with it. Closer to home, the Alzheimer Society of Canada tells us that the number of Canadians living with cognitive impairment now stands at 747,000. That number is expected to double to 1.4 million by 2031. These numbers include not only those Canadians diagnosed with various forms of dementia — including Alzheimer's — but also those showing signs of cognitive impairment, a condition that often leads to other forms of dementia. Further, it's estimated that Alzheimer's — the most common type of dementia, affecting memory, thinking, and behaviour — is currently costing us between $150 billion to $200 billion per year globally. That's more than it costs to deal with cancer and heart disease combined, believe it or not. Surprisingly, the biggest cost isn't the money spent on drugs or medical treatment, it's the cost of providing the personal care for those who're mentally impaired and can no longer look after themselves.

To understand the sort of impact this will have on society — and is having, right now — you should know that, in 2011, individual family members in Canada spent 444 million *unpaid* hours looking after someone suffering from dementia. We're talking about in one year, folks. To break this down even further, those 444 million unpaid hours represent more than a quarter of a million full-time equivalent employees lost to the workforce, and $11 billion in lost income. In less than twenty-five years, we'll likely be investing 1.2 billion unpaid hours per year in order to look after those loved ones who can no longer look after themselves. Estimates suggest that the combined direct (medical) and indirect (lost earnings) costs of dealing with dementia in Canada come out to $33 billion a year. This is expected to rise to $293 billion by the year 2040. And yet, despite all the evidence, while thirteen countries around the world have established a national dementia plan, Canada is not one of them. You have to wonder why.

I have a theory or two.

For one thing, dementia — and, in particular, Alzheimer's — is not a "sexy" disease. Let's face it, no matter how skilled a photographer or videographer you find to create a campaign, no one's going to want to see an advertisement featuring a mentally challenged grandpa or horribly agitated grandma. The other problem is that while politicians love photo ops — they want to be seen doing something good by as many members of the public as possible, especially if it involves handing out our tax dollars — no token amount of money is going to hold back the tide of this epidemic. It's going to take a real commitment, one few have the guts to make.

Unfortunately, if someone doesn't soon step forward and show some real leadership here, then this third health care tsunami could well turn into a mega-tsunami — one that threatens to bankrupt us and strip away the very fabric of our society, drowning us in a wave of sorrow and regret. We can't afford to bury our collective heads in the sand and pretend this isn't happening. We must act now before it's too late.

Luckily, there is hope. Remember the boomers and zoomers I spoke about earlier? They're the ones who'll ultimately step in and save the day. With this group's accumulated wealth, its refusal to accept wait-lists or mediocrity, and its disdain for know-nothing, do-nothing elected officials, those born during the two decades following the Second World War will drive the agenda and ensure something is indeed done to prepare for the aforementioned three health care tsunamis that are waiting to wipe us out. In the same way they have embraced life and refused to let physical infirmities slow them down, I believe the boomers — and especially the zoomers — will demand governments of all political stripes come up with not just a strategy for dealing with obesity and diabetes but also one for dementia, particularly Alzheimer's. They'll insist that resources be invested not only in research, but also in helping families deal with the high costs of caring for those who're battling obesity, diabetes, and dementia. It *can* be done but only if everyone is willing to join in and not leave the heavy lifting to just a select few.

THE HYPOCRITICAL OATH

To be brutally frank, before I came to work at the Ontario Medical Association in the spring of 1995, I didn't have an especially high opinion of doctors. Oh, sure, I liked my own doctor just fine. Dr. David Grotell, a general practitioner specializing in hypnotherapy, worked out of a medium-sized clinic in Toronto's west end. I'd originally been referred to him by my mother's doctor in hopes that he'd be able to do something about my migraine headaches. Dr. Grotell's calm, patient approach proved helpful, and I learned to keep the headaches under control without resorting to medication — medication that had previously packed an extra thirty pounds on me in little more than a month in the early 1980s. I was so pleased with the results, and with the new lease on life hypnotherapy had given me, I asked Dr. Grotell if he'd consider becoming my family doctor. He said yes and continued in that role for the next two decades.

Organized medicine, however ... well, that was a different story. Having lived through the doctors' strike in Ontario in 1986, watching the leadership of the OMA lose a most winnable battle and flushing its credibility and that of its members down the drain at the same time, I couldn't help feeling those so-called fat cats, as the *Toronto Star* and other media outlets liked to portray doctors, had got what they'd deserved. Like many Ontarians, I was part of that great silent majority who delighted in seeing David Peterson and his new Liberal government stick it to the medical profession.

But my attitude soon changed. Doctors, I discovered shortly after I began working for them, were not at all the way they'd been depicted in the media. As someone — it might have been Dr. Michael Thoburn, former OMA president and director of professional services — explained to me, "Being a doctor isn't what you do, it's what you are." Or to put it another way, for these folks, medicine isn't just a job, it's a calling, much like the priesthood. Being a physician is an honourable profession, one that attracts not only the best and the brightest, but also the caring and the giving.

Regrettably, we, as patients, have stood idly by while our elected officials, spurred on by other stakeholders, have taken baseball bats — disguised as legislation — and swung away at the medical profession as if it were a giant piñata. Whether we're talking about the outlawing of extra-billing by David Peterson in 1986; the "deal with the Devil" made by Bob Rae in 1991, offering the Ontario Medical Association the right to Rand the province's doctors in lieu of a fee increase; the granting of Kafkaesque powers to the College of Physicians and Surgeons of Ontario's Medical Review Committee by Mike Harris in 1996; or the recent ham-handed attempts by federal finance minister Bill Morneau to reform our tax system by changing the rules, primarily at the expense of physicians, for small businesses that have chosen to incorporate, politicians of all political stripes have undoubtedly had it in for doctors.

What makes these actions even worse, in my mind anyhow, is the cynical way in which those we favoured with our vote and trusted to do the right thing have actually put all of us in danger by dumping on doctors and engaging in a most dangerous game. For, you see, doctors are a special breed. They are like the workhorse or the mule — they will keep their heads down and continue to work the plow, no matter how many times you beat and abuse them.

This is why, now that we have reached the midpoint of our journey together, I feel it would be a good idea to pause for a moment or two and turn the spotlight on physicians and their relationship with their political masters. I plan on examining three things specifically. First, doctors and the Stockholm Syndrome. Because of their psychological makeup — all the things that go into creating the kind of person who'd want to be a physician in the first place — doctors exhibit a disturbing tendency to, if not actually fall in love with their abusers, show a willingness to forgive those who treat them so badly. Next, I want to share with you the story of Dr. Anthony Hsu, the Welland, Ontario, pediatrician who was audited to death by the CPSO's Medical Review Committee in 2003. Dr. Hsu, a kind and gentle man, committed suicide after cashing in his RRSPs so that he could reimburse the Ontario government the more than $100,000 they'd extorted from him. Finally, I plan on looking at a relatively new phenomenon, something I like to call "Dr. Health Minister." I will carefully examine the actions of former Ontario health minister Dr. Eric Hoskins and former federal health minister Jane Philpott — two medical doctors turned public servants turned professional assassins.

Doctors and the Stockholm Syndrome

On August 23, 1973, a thirty-two-year-old career criminal by the name of Jan-Erik Olsson, who had just escaped from prison, entered a bank in Stockholm, Sweden, along with an accomplice, and began firing off his machine gun, announcing to a group of startled bank employees, "The party has just begun!" The employees had sticks of dynamite strapped to their bodies and were held hostage until they were finally rescued five days later.

What makes this story particularly fascinating — to me and to a number of psychologists who've studied other hostage-taking scenarios — is the rather shocking and totally unexpected attitude the hostages exhibited following their release. In media interview after media interview, all four of the hostages showed support for their captors and empathized with them. Even more bizarrely, the bank employees were fearful of those who'd come to their rescue, believing irrationally that the robbers were actually *protecting* them from the police. During a phone call from the vault with Sweden's prime minister, one of the captives even implored the PM to provide a getaway car so the hostages could leave the bank along with the kidnappers.

"So, what does all this have to do with doctors?" you're probably wondering.

Good question. Let me try to provide an answer. Having worked closely with physicians for the past quarter-century, I've come to know how doctors think, behave, and react. Believe me when I say that those who heal us are not like you and me. They're not motivated by greed or money. They don't believe in playing politics or getting even. And they most certainly aren't trying to win any popularity contests by doing the politically expedient thing instead of the right thing. Doctors, for the most part, are solid citizens. We can trust them. We can put our faith in them. And, unlike our elected officials, we can *believe* what they tell us. But doctors are not perfect ... far from it. They're gullible and easily fooled. Time and time again, they make bad business decisions and often put their faith in the wrong people. Worst of all, they'll go to almost any lengths to make excuses for those in charge — even when those same politicians are threatening both their livelihoods and their lives.

That doctors here in Canada are suffering from a severe case of Stockholm Syndrome there can be no doubt. To prove this, I'm going to share with you some more inside information that's not generally known to the public. We're going to have to travel all the way back to 1994 — the year before Mike Harris and his Progressive Conservative Party tried to bring common sense to Ontario. In 1994, Dr. Hugh Scully and a group of prominent Ontario doctors produced a report that called for, among other things, a parallel private health care system. You heard me right. The hybrid health care system that I and others are so vocally advocating for had its beginnings in the Scully Report. As previously mentioned, three months after I began working at the Ontario Medical Association, Harris and his fellow common sense revolutionaries surprised just about everyone by winning a majority, defeating both the Liberals and the NDP by a wide margin. Within the OMA, there was a great deal of debate as to when would be the right time to present the new premier with his own copy of the Scully Report.

Just as Rome burned while Nero fiddled, however, things were happening behind the scenes, and voila, before anyone knew what was happening, finance minister Ernie Eves stood in the legislature and introduced the Savings and Restructuring Act — an enabling piece of legislation that would, in effect, give several ministers, including the newly installed health minister Jim Wilson, the right to play God. We've already examined this particular act in some detail. One thing that's not generally known is that in the original version of the bill the Ontario Medical Association was going to be legislated out of existence. The new government also stated they would no longer cover any portion of doctors' malpractice insurance fees.

Following a series of very public skirmishes, including a rather effective job action undertaken by the province's obstetricians and gynecologists, who refused to take on any more pregnant patients unless the government changed its mind about their malpractice insurance fees, the OMA and the Harris government eventually hammered out a new Physician Services Agreement in 1997 — one that would allow the medical profession to "co-manage" Ontario's health care system through the Physician Services Committee.

This was it, right there. The moment when things could have gone one way, but instead went the other. Doctors, beaten and abused and obviously worn out, caved in and agreed to help fix health care by co-managing the system. I remember the sense of jubilation inside OMA headquarters. Everyone there — including me, I'll admit — thought we'd actually pulled off something of a coup. Co-managing Ontario's health care system. Wow! What more could you ask for — especially if you were a special interest group like the Ontario Medical Association? Unfortunately, as we saw with those Stockholm bank employees, snuggling up with those who may not have your best interests at heart is a poor idea at best and a dangerous one at worst. For not only would the province's doctors do everyone a huge disservice in the years to come by propping up our crumbling health care system so our elected officials could continue to perpetrate the myth that our country has the best system in the world, they also fell asleep at the switch and failed to realize they were being recruited by the Harris government to weed out fraud — something Jim Wilson was obsessed with. Thus, when the CPSO's Medical Review Committee began ramping up its activities in 1999, the OMA turned a blind eye to what was going on, assuming that if their partners in managing the health care system felt doctors were guilty of ripping off the system, then those doctors must indeed be guilty.

Audited to Death

To fully appreciate the insidiousness of what happened to Dr. Anthony "Tony" Hsu, we must once again go back in time to the early 1990s. Fearful of hitting the debt wall — a level of government indebtedness that would result in bankers refusing to lend more money, a situation that would leave, in this case, the Province of Ontario no choice but to declare bankruptcy — the Bob Rae government "negotiated" something called the social contract with a number of stakeholders. Much to everyone's surprise, the Ontario Medical Association agreed to a 10 percent clawback on fees paid to its members — every tenth patient a doctor treated would be for free.

The OMA, having recently been guaranteed millions of dollars in annual membership dues thanks to the Ontario Medical Association Dues Act, which was passed by the NDP in 1991, was somehow able to convince its members that subsidizing the province's health care system in order to help bail out the fiscally challenged government was a good idea. For their part, doctors, having been taken hostage by their own representative every bit as much as by the government, reluctantly agreed.

Shortly after the surprise election of Mike Harris on June 8, 1995, the clawbacks came to an end. But at the same time, it seems those who had now taken hold of the reins of power came up with a new idea. Although I can't prove it, I suspect that one of Harris's advisors, perhaps aided by a ministry of health civil servant, floated the idea of *scaring* the province's doctors into clawing back their own fees by threatening them with the CPSO's Medical Review Committee. By granting the MRC new powers through the soon-to-be-introduced Savings and Restructuring Act, the government would have the ability to keep a lid on rising health care costs by scaring physicians into under-billing. Thus began a witch hunt unlike any seen in Ontario before or since.

As with the AIDS epidemic in the mid-1980s, it wasn't clear at first what was happening. MRC inspectors would send individual doctors a letter, telling them they were suspected of inappropriate billing. The inspectors — fellow doctors, who'd been hired by the college to conduct these "investigations" into the billing practices of their colleagues — would then arrive at the physician's office, demanding to see confidential patient files. Typically, the inspectors would leave with a hundred or so files, telling the shell-shocked doctor that they'd hear from them in a couple of weeks. A month or so later, another letter would arrive, informing the victimized doctor that the one hundred files showed they'd over-billed the health care system by $10,000. Since the doctor had one thousand patients, it stood to reason — according to the messed-up logic of the MRC — they must have been over-billing for all those patients, as well, and therefore owed the government something on the order of $100,000.

Doctors were given the option to pay up right away or request a hearing. However, the individual doctor needed to know they'd be responsible for covering the cost of the hearing — typically $30,000 or more — as well as any interest accrued while awaiting the outcome of the hearing. In other words, doctors were found guilty and had to pay for the right to prove their innocence. Needless to say, this was not natural justice — it was a *perversion* of justice. Many doctors chose to forgo the hearing and quietly pay the penalty in hopes this Kafkaesque nightmare might soon be over. Others fought against what many felt was government-sponsored extortion and had their penalties reduced. As for the Ontario Medical Association, it did its best to ignore what was going on.

Not surprisingly, those Oz-like creatures lurking in the shadows pulling switches were pleased at how well their scheme was working. But that's when they made their first mistake. They got greedy and started targeting *groups* of doctors. Neurologists. General practitioners. Pediatricians.

This is how Tony Hsu became ensnared.

Dr. Hsu was a busy pediatrician based in Welland, Ontario. He was well liked, extremely gifted, and truly cared about his patients. Like many of his colleagues, Dr. Hsu was so overwhelmed by the number of children he was looking after that he often took shortcuts when filling out patient charts. For instance, instead of writing down what he didn't find when he examined a child, Tony would only write down what he *did* discover. In this way, he was able to spend more time seeing patients and less time on paperwork. Now, to any normal person, Dr. Hsu's approach to patient care would seem like a sensible one. He put his patients first and didn't allow himself to drown in a whirlpool of bureaucracy. The MRC, though, didn't see it that way. To them, Dr. Anthony Hsu was a thief, a bad doctor who was ripping off the system and bringing shame to his profession — all because the government's computer showed Dr. Hsu billed more annual checkups than the average pediatrician (even though he also billed one-third less consultation fees, which saved the health care system tens of thousands of dollars, something the MRC failed to share, interested as they were in only portraying him as guilty). Once they were done with the poor man, Tony — his life shattered and his reputation in tatters — walked into Lake Ontario, humiliated and defeated. His body washed up onshore about a week later, not far from where his abandoned car had been discovered.

I remember seeing Dr. Hsu seated in the public gallery of the Queen's Park media studio in January 2003, where Dr. Farouk Dindar and other members of the newly formed Ontario Doctors for Fair Audits group were holding a media conference, before taking their protest to the front steps of the College of Physicians and Surgeons of Ontario a couple of blocks away. Dr. Hsu had recently cashed in his RRSP in order to pay back the money — $108,162 to be exact — the MRC said he owed the Government of Ontario. I've never seen anyone look so vulnerable in all my life. I'll always regret not having gone up to Dr. Hsu to tell him what a hero I thought he was for breaking the silence and speaking up about the unfairness of what had happened to him.

It was shortly after the media conference that Tony made his lonely drive to Vineland — alone — where he walked away from his car and ended his life.

Not surprisingly, Dr. Hsu's suicide was the turning point in the battle to put an end to the MRC's reign of terror. NDP MPP Peter Kormos joined together with Dr. Douglas Mark of the Coalition of Family Physicians of Ontario (now DoctorsOntario) and members of Ontario Doctors for Fair Audits to demand that newly installed health minister George Smitherman do something about the draconian changes made to the province's OHIP audit system by the Progressive Conservative government in 1999. In short order, retired Supreme Court of Canada Justice Peter Cory was appointed by Smitherman to conduct an inquiry into the activities of the MRC. And a moratorium was placed on further audits until Justice Cory could make his recommendations.

During Justice Cory's inquiry, the disturbing case of Dr. Brian Lyttle came to light. Lyttle, a London, Ontario, pediatric respirologist, was ordered to repay the Ontario Health Insurance Plan thousands of dollars because — get this — he failed to conduct rectal or gynecological assessments on his young patients while he examined them. As another pediatrician remarked to Justice Cory, referring to the Lyttle case, "Imagine bringing your four-year-old girl to me for a cough and I do a rectal or vaginal exam. I'd be hauled up before the College of Physicians and Surgeons' disciplinary committee for professional misconduct before you could say 'Jack Robinson.'"

Dr. Lyttle appealed the Medical Review Committee's decision to the Health Services Appeal and Review Board, which found that the MRC's interpretation was wrong and ordered Dr. Lyttle be reimbursed in full. "In this instance," Justice Cory stated, "the young patient did not require, nor did the physician conduct, a vaginal examination." And yet, the government insisted the MRC's procedures met the requirements of, and were satisfied that their process met the definition of, natural justice (i.e., the accused is presumed innocent until found guilty). "In my view," the judge wrote in his final report, with just a hint of sarcasm, "one would not want the process to 'work' in that fashion too often."

Shortly after Justice Cory made his recommendations, and Minister Smitherman introduced a new piece of legislation — the Health System Improvements Act — which effectively drove a stake through the heart of the MRC, I was invited to lunch by Tony's widow, Irene Hsu. More than perhaps any other single person or organization, Irene had been responsible for righting this wrong, saving countless other doctors from suffering the same fate as her husband. At the end of our lunch, Irene surprised me by presenting me with a beautiful porcelain tiger. I still keep that tiger at my desk, on a shelf just above my computer. Whenever I am stuck and in need of inspiration I look up and see the tiger and remember the many heroes responsible for the dismantling of the Medical Review Committee — especially Tony and Irene. Two tigers who fought the good fight — with incredible courage and class — right up until the end.

Dr. Health Minister: A New Phenomenon

One of my key responsibilities during the time I spent with the Ontario Medical Association was to encourage physicians to become more politically active. Together with the chair of the OMA's political action committee, Dr. Albert Schumacher, we set up the MD/MPP program, which was designed to assist doctors in lobbying their local elected representatives at the grassroots level. We also developed and launched an event that eventually became an annual tradition at Queen's Park, called appropriately enough "Doctor Day." But it was a third initiative — which we dubbed the MD Candidate program — that took political action to a whole other level.

Bringing in some of the top Canadian political operatives of the day, we worked with doctors, their spouses, and their siblings to develop an impressive roster of potential candidates. Not only did we prepare them for a life in politics, we also liaised with all three political parties in Ontario — the Progressive Conservatives, the Liberals, and the New Democrats — to help smooth the way, when it came time, for our MD candidates to try to secure a nomination. No expense was spared, as Dr. Schumacher and I regularly brought a dozen or so doctors and staff with us on our yearly pilgrimage to Washington, D.C., so that our people could attend the three-day training sessions put on by the Campaigns & Elections group.

The main reason the OMA was so keen on encouraging doctors to run for public office, I suspect, is because, historically, the medical profession was often ignored when big decisions — especially those about health care and finance — were being made. And while it's true Dr. Charles Tupper, the former premier of Nova Scotia and one of the Fathers of Confederation, served as prime minister of Canada — only for ten weeks, however — physicians were sorely lacking a place at the table. For instance, until Dr. Jane Philpott was named minister of health by Prime Minister Justin Trudeau in November of 2015, no doctor had ever served in that capacity at the federal level. In Ontario, it was much the same. Until Dr. Eric Hoskins became minister of health and long-term care in June of 2014, no doctor had been in charge of the health care portfolio since Dr. Matthew Dymond, who'd held the post for nearly eleven years, from 1958 to 1969.

While the naming of Dr. Philpott and Dr. Hoskins should have been a cause for much rejoicing and celebration among the medical community, it didn't quite work out that way. Whether these two talented and seemingly capable physicians underwent some kind of conversion on the road to Damascus or were simply good at disguising the fact they were both, in reality, wolves in sheep's clothing, we'll never know. Suffice to say, these two doctors have done more harm to Canada's medical profession — and, by extension, to our health care system — than almost any other health ministers, either federally or provincially.

Let's start with Dr. Hoskins. While I acknowledge the good doctor inherited a mess from his predecessor, Deb Matthews, as a result of her unilaterally making a number of reckless and irresponsible cuts to the fee schedule — cuts that put patient care at risk and pushed some of Ontario's physicians closer to the edge of bankruptcy — the sad truth is that Minister Hoskins seemingly took great delight in pouring gasoline on the fire and fanning the flames by suggesting his colleagues were greedy and only interested in money. As if that wasn't bad enough, he took to the airwaves, as well as incorporating the latest social media tools, to conduct his alarming and disheartening campaign of disinformation. Even worse, he took advantage of the fact he was a physician, and hence much more trusted by the public than your average run-of-the-mill politician. Time and time again, Dr. Hoskins made it clear he — *and he alone* — knew how to fix our health care system, and that he was quite prepared to do it with or without the help of other doctors.

Needless to say, the health minister's approach definitely *wasn't* what the doctor had ordered. I was personally so concerned about Dr. Hoskins's approach that I made a complaint to the CPSO's Medical Review Committee — yes, the same Medical Review Committee that had been responsible for the demise of Dr. Hsu. Although the MRC did, to their credit, conduct a thorough review of the health minister's actions and public pronouncements, they let him off the hook because he claimed he was no longer a doctor — he was now a politician and, therefore, not subject to the rules and regulations governing his colleagues.

I kid you not.

While Dr. Hoskins has shown himself to be no friend of physicians, Dr. Philpott, in many ways, has proven herself to be even worse. Speaking at the Canadian Medical Association's 150th annual meeting in the summer of 2017, shortly after federal finance minister Bill Morneau announced he was making changes to the way small-business owners were allowed to incorporate their businesses in order to save for retirement and pay less taxes — changes which would negatively impact thousands of physicians all across Canada, many of whom had been encouraged to incorporate in lieu of a fee increase — Dr. Philpott had the audacity to suggest doctors would've had nothing to be concerned about if they'd only bothered to *read* Minister Morneau's proposals. Now, if there's one thing I know about doctors — remember, there isn't a doctor practising in this country who doesn't, rightly or wrongly, fancy himself or herself as something of an expert in the field of law — they *all* would've read Bill Morneau's proposals. Not just once. Not just twice. But three times.

As if this wasn't bad enough, Dr. Philpott — speaking from the bully pulpit she'd constructed for herself — then suggested that doctors should use their unique position in society to help the less fortunate. "Because you are a doctor," Minister Philpott said, "society has granted you power and privilege, respect and responsibility. There is no better use of that power than to advocate on behalf of those who do not have the same opportunities."

Oh, give me a break. I mean, really. This is just the sort of social engineering BS that seems to have invaded the corridors of power everywhere in this country — from coast to coast to coast.

The champagne socialists who find themselves in charge in the twenty-first century seem to think every successful Canadian entrepreneur must be so overwhelmed by guilt that they can't give away their fortune fast enough. No wonder Dr. Philpott was so quick to throw her colleagues under the bus and support the finance minister's ill-conceived tax reform plan. The health minister took it a step further, mothballing her own incorporated practice about a week or so after Bill Morneau's proposals became public. Her excuse for doing so? Like Dr. Hoskins, Minister Philpott intimated that she, too, was now a politician and not a doctor.

As someone who has devoted a sizeable chunk of his life to helping physicians become more politically active, and even getting doctors elected at all three levels of government, I can't begin to tell you how disgusted I am at the hypocrisy displayed by the likes of Dr. Hoskins and Dr. Philpott. They both made the clear and deliberate choice to put themselves first, ahead of their colleagues and their patients. Or to put it another way, they're not doctors — they're *politicians*. No one with an ounce of sense would ever believe a word coming out of the mouth of either one of them.

We can only hope that someday soon a doctor-politician will emerge who's willing to be honest and tell the truth, one who knows what needs to be done to save Canada's health care system, and who'll stop at nothing to ensure we move beyond the status quo and embrace the future — whatever it may hold for us — clear-eyed, clear-headed, and pure of heart. What a change that would be from the likes of Drs. Hoskins and Philpott and their obscene adherence to the Hypocritical Oath.

PART III
FIRST, DO NO HARM

Sex, politics, and religion. These are the three things I'm told you should never talk about in mixed company. In addition to this troika of taboo topics, I've recently discovered a fourth: health care. You heard me right. *Health care.* Honestly, tossing a grenade into a room full of pacifists couldn't create more chaos than announcing publicly you're in favour of a hybrid health care system and that it's high time Canada embraced the future instead of clinging pathetically to the past. I made this surprising discovery while chatting with some people — strangers, mostly — at a friend's place. We'd gathered to celebrate his wife's birthday and were doing so in style, roasting a pig and eating corn on the cob. My friend mentioned I'm a rather vocal advocate for private health care when he introduced me upon my arrival. One of those in attendance — an American who'd become a Canadian citizen after having spent the past forty-plus years living in Toronto — wanted to know what I had against our free health care system.

"For one thing," I replied, "it's not free. For another, it's not much of a system."

The man took umbrage with my comments and began telling me about his experience with Canada's "jewel" of a health care system. "I had a heart attack last year," he said. "Would've died if it hadn't been for the doctors and nurses on duty in the emergency department that day. They saved my life. And it didn't cost me a nickel!"

I smiled and said I was glad to hear that. He clearly was one of the lucky ones. So much luckier that the sixty-three thousand Canadians who'd had to leave the country the previous year and go elsewhere because they couldn't afford to wait any longer for medical treatment. The man scoffed at this, called it "right-wing propaganda," and said I was just like all the others, running down the best health care system in the world just because my rich friends and I wanted to push people like him out of the way and jump the queue.

"Not so," I said. "First of all, I'm not rich. I'm middle class — just like you. And secondly, if I was rich, I wouldn't need another, private tier of health care. I'd just hop on a plane and fly to the States."

I then took the opportunity to point out that Canada, while it once *did* have the best health care system in the world, can no longer make that boast. Study after study shows our system is in decline, that wait-lists for procedures are growing and people are dying because governments of all political stripes have been forced to take an axe to medicare, cutting funding and programs in an insane attempt to prove our unsustainable health care system is somehow sustainable, that the status quo is just fine. The Supreme Court of Canada was pretty clear in 2005, I added, when they rendered a decision in the Chaoulli case. "Access to a wait list is not access to health care," as one of the judges said.

The man took a sip of his drink and replied, "All I know is I'm glad I don't live in America anymore. The last thing I'd want is to have to deal with their messed-up system."

I told him I agreed but that, unfortunately, unless our elected officials stop trying to distract us with fairy tales and finally come clean, I'm afraid we're going to end up with the very thing everyone says they don't want — namely, a health care system that looks a whole lot like the one in the States.

"So, what's your solution?" the man asked.

"We need a made-in-Canada hybrid health care system," I replied. "One that takes the best elements of other health care systems throughout the world and blends them — in creative and courageous ways — so that we might ultimately come out of the other end with a real health care *system*, one that treats the whole person and not just the illness. A system that isn't simply an insurance scheme, but one that allows patients to take charge of their own medical care, paying for what they want, without being forced to travel abroad to receive medical treatment. This is my dream.

"Sadly," I told the man, "neither you nor I are likely to live long enough to see the day when that dream becomes a reality. So long as politicians continue to wrap themselves in the flag of medicare and declare they'll defend Canada's health care system to the bitter end, I'm afraid we're doomed to stand hopelessly by and watch more of our fellow citizens suffer — and yes, even die — on wait-lists, while those in charge ration health care and deny us our rights and freedoms."

"We're being played," I sighed. "This madness has to stop … and soon."

•••

Change has to happen, there's no denying it … on that, most everyone agrees. But it's crucial when changing things that care is taken to ensure the new system will be better than the one it's replacing, that in improving one thing you don't inadvertently make something else worse. This part of the book is called "First, Do No Harm," but I could've just as easily named it "The Law of Unintended Consequences." Over the last few years, governments across Canada have initiated changes in their health care systems in order to improve them. At least, that was the intent. As we'll see, though, the best laid plans often go astray. In this section, we'll take a look at a number of government initiatives — the increased use of midwives and nurse practitioners, primary care reform, electronic medical records, the Transformation Agenda, and Choosing Wisely — all of which, one way or another, have created some serious unintended consequences for us to deal with.

•••

Before we carry on with this part of our journey, however, I think it would be worth it to pause for a few moments and talk about the law of unintended consequences.

While the concept of unintended consequences was first put forth by John Locke and Adam Smith many moons ago, it was sociologist Robert K.

Merton who popularized the term in his 1936 paper, "The Unanticipated Consequences of Purposive Social Action." Merton listed the following five possible causes of unintended consequences in his paper: ignorance, errors in analyzing the problem, immediate interests overriding long-term interests, basic values, and self-defeating prophecy. In modern times, the law of unintended consequences has been used as a warning for those who would stick their noses where they don't belong. A perfect example of this would be the Ontario Liberals' decision to phase out coal plants in favour of green energy — a decision that has led to hydro bills in the province more than doubling over the past decade, details of which were contained in a 2015 report by the province's auditor general.

But lest you think it's only the team in red that's made mistakes, both the Ontario New Democrats and Progressive Conservatives should hang their collective heads in shame, as well, over some awfully bad decisions they've made during the past thirty-plus years:

- *Premier Bob Rae cuts medical school enrolment by 10 percent in 1992:* Hard to say if this was the dumbest decision ever made by an elected official but it definitely ranks right up there. The Rae government, desperate for cash to help keep a $10 billion deficit from rising even higher, decided that since doctors cost the health care system so much money, the only course of action available to the government was to reduce the number of doctors by cutting medical school enrolment by 10 percent. Even though his own advisors told him it was a bad idea, with serious long-term consequences, Premier Rae went ahead and did it anyway. As a result, millions of Ontarians have been left without a family doctor — a problem we're still trying to rectify nearly thirty years later.
- *Premier Mike Harris closes hospitals in 1996:* Granted, Ontario's health care system was in definite need of restructuring when Mike Harris took over as premier in 1995. Unfortunately, his bull-in-a-china-shop approach to closing and amalgamating hospitals caused more problems than it solved. Worse, failing to deal with the *real* problem — a lack of long-term beds for seniors

and those who couldn't be cared for at home — led to overcrowding in hospital emergency departments. As we've recently witnessed in Ottawa and other places, where local hospitals are operating at 120 percent capacity, forcing them to stick sick patients in hallways and broom closets, Premier Harris also failed to get it right. This is a shame, because his plan could have worked had the Progressive Conservative leader been more conciliatory and less confrontational in his approach.

These two premiers have nothing on David Peterson, though, who surely deserves to be a charter member in the Law of Unintended Consequences Hall of Fame for the following smooth move:

- *Premier David Peterson bans "balance billing" in 1986:* Believe it or not, Ontario's health care system wasn't always the mess it is today. Before the introduction of the Canada Health Act in 1983, things worked rather well — in no small part because the Province of Ontario allowed balance billing. Doctors had the option of charging patients the difference between the Ontario Medical Association fee schedule and what the Ontario Health Insurance Plan was willing to cover. In the mid-1980s, that difference was roughly 10 percent. Today, it's more than 50 percent. The Peterson government, by convincing the public that doctors were "extra" billing, managed to pass legislation outlawing the practice — thereby removing an important safety valve that had, up until then, ensured the system was sustainable.

As American economist and Nobel Prize winner Milton Friedman so succinctly put it, "One of the great mistakes is to judge policies and programs by their intentions rather than their results."

Pretty much sums it up.

Midwives and Nurse Practitioners

Full disclosure: I've spent most of the past two decades fighting the good fight on behalf of doctors, as their lobbyist, strategist, and advisor. Although I have contracted to work as a consultant for other health care groups — the Registered Nurses' Association of Ontario and the Ontario Kinesiology Association are two that come to mind — most of the work I've done in the health care field has been in the service of physicians. So, it will come as no surprise that I'm not a fan of either midwives or nurse practitioners.

Now, before you go accusing me of being a misogynist, I need to point out that my misgivings have nothing to do with the fact there are a great many more women working in these two professions than men. No, my concerns are based on the fact that politicians — having so badly mismanaged our precious health care resources, as well as choking off the supply of doctors in the early 1990s and vilifying those doctors still practising in the subsequent decades — have tried to mask their mistakes by pretending midwives and nurse practitioners are somehow an acceptable solution to our current doctor shortage. As Dr. David Bridgeo, chair of the OMA section on general and family practice, quipped, "Having these roles filled by non-medical personnel is like having a member of the flight crew fly the plane." Or to put it another way, it's like insisting a flight attendant can handle everything a pilot can — with the exception of takeoffs and landings.

Midwifery, of course, is a very old practice, dating back to ancient Egypt. While many women prefer this option to giving birth in a hospital under the care of an OB-GYN, the fact is engaging a midwife not only presents a significant number of risks, it also costs our health care system a lot more money.

Unlike doctors, midwives enjoy a salary and benefits, have a pension, and receive vacation pay. They don't have to shell out any money for an office or equipment — the government provides all that for them — nor are they responsible for the cost of malpractice insurance. Even worse, when a midwife encounters a problem — known in medical circles as a "difficult" birth — they call in a doctor, who then takes over the case and often must perform a Caesarean section in order to guarantee the safety of both the mother and the newborn.

Doctors, on the other hand, are on the hook for their own malpractice insurance (although some form of rebate has typically been negotiated with government over the past few decades, there is no guarantee future governments will continue to do so), must cover the cost of their own office and equipment, receive no salary or benefits, and don't get a pension or vacation pay. As well, they're the ones who get called in at the eleventh hour to save the day when something goes wrong and the midwife needs help because he or she doesn't have the necessary training to manage difficult cases in the same manner as a doctor.

The playing field for nurse practitioners isn't particularly level either. While the McGuinty government in Ontario originally promised that nurse practitioners wouldn't be allowed to run their own clinics and would instead have to work under the supervision of a doctor, in no time at all nurse practitioner–led clinics began to pop up around the province — mostly in the northern part of Ontario, where doctor shortages are especially severe. As if this wasn't bad enough, thanks to a relentless lobbying campaign by Doris Grinspun and the Registered Nurses' Association of Ontario, the government soon agreed to expand the powers of nurse practitioners, allowing them to prescribe a wide range of drugs, as well as ordering X-rays and CT scans. What makes this especially galling — not just to doctors but also to veteran health care observers such as myself — is that our elected officials are once again playing politics with our health care system by pretending the doctor shortage they caused can be solved by replacing physicians with health care providers who simply haven't had the same amount of education and training as doctors.

To suggest, as some have done, that a nurse practitioner can provide the same level of care as a doctor is just plain dishonest. And yet, for thousands of Ontarians who've been without a family doctor for years and have little chance of finding one because of where they live, having a nurse practitioner is better than nothing — even though it's in no way an adequate substitute for a doctor.

So, what should government do in order to deal with our alarming shortage of physicians? Three things: (1) increase medical school enrolment by 10 percent; (2) make it easier for young doctors to find a training position once they've graduated — our current system of matching recently graduated doctors with the right medical residency program clearly isn't working, as illustrated by the appalling suicide of Dr. Robert Chu, a bright and promising medical student who was trapped in a system where provincial governments control the number of residency positions and denied him the right to continue his career (and have any kind of shot of paying off his massive student debt) for reasons that make sense to no one; and (3) embrace the concept of physician assistants (also known as physician extenders).

Let's take a look at each of these in a little more detail.

We've already seen what can happen when desperate politicians make bad decisions based on the latest polling numbers. The fallout from former premier Bob Rae's decision back in 1992 to reduce medical school enrolment by 10 percent is arguably still being felt today. Hopefully, newly elected Ontario premier Doug Ford will show a little leadership on the issue, and, instead of cutting medical school enrolment, will increase it by 10 percent or more. This would go a long way toward ensuring future generations of Ontarians will not only be able to find a family doctor but will also be able to better access a specialist when they need one.

Increasing medical school enrolment by itself, however, will not be enough if we don't fix what is obviously a badly broken medical residency matching program that governs people like Dr. Chu. It's estimated to cost taxpayers half a million dollars to train a doctor — this in addition to the $100,000 to $150,000 of personal debt each medical student is forced to run up to finish their degree. Why would we then put our investment at risk by allowing the luck of the draw to determine if and when a young doctor might be assigned a spot to continue his or her medical training? Doctors already have the highest suicide rate among all professionals. Why add to their burden by allowing a flawed system to continue to ruin lives and flush taxpayers' dollars down the drain?

Perhaps the best thing our elected officials could do to show they're serious about helping physicians do their job would be to get behind the concept of physician assistants in a big way. No idea in the past few years has shown such potential to help alleviate Canada's doctor shortage problem. Working closely with doctors, physician assistants — or PAs, as they're more commonly referred to — allow doctors to spend more time actually dealing with patients and less time drowning in a never-ending sea of red tape and paperwork. By "extending" what a regular doctor can do, physician assistants are able to provide the doctors they work side by side with, with the most valuable commodity of all — time. Although a relatively new concept in Canada — currently, there are about three hundred PAs in practice in this country — physician assistants are extremely popular elsewhere. For example, there are more than seventy thousand physician assistants in the United States, working right alongside doctors in both primary care practice settings and various specialties.

Bottom line: There's no easy way to train someone for a career in medicine. There are no shortcuts. There are no substitutes. While midwives and nurse practitioners can be *part* of the solution, they're definitely not *the* solution. Anyone who tells you anything different is simply talking out of their hat.

Primary Care Reform

Shortly after I was hired by the Ontario Medical Association in the spring of 1995, I became aware of the term "primary care reform." I can't remember whether I first heard about primary care reform during a board meeting, a political action committee meeting, or my first OMA council meeting, which took place in late May, just days before Mike Harris and the Progressive Conservative Party swept into power. In all likelihood, it was during that first council, which I was expected to sit through as a new hire in hopes that I might learn something about medical politics — if only through osmosis.

At some point during that two-day meeting, Dr. Wendy Graham, a family doctor who resided and practised in North Bay, Ontario — coincidentally, the same city Mike Harris lived in — took to the stage and shared her thoughts on how Ontario might reform primary care in order to help family doctors and general practitioners, who were struggling to adequately serve their patients while paying the bills and saddled with what Dr. Graham and others considered to be an outdated fee-for-service model. Dr. Graham spoke about "baskets of services," "bundles," "shadow billing," and "rostering." Being a newbie, I hadn't a clue about any of this, but over the next couple of decades I'd not only come to understand why primary care was so badly in need of reform, I'd also play a not-insignificant — if behind-the-scenes — role in helping the Harris government launch even more pilot projects for what would come to be known as the "alphabet soup" of primary care models.

Before I take you there, I want to explain why primary care has been so hard to reform in Canada in the first place. For the most part, it harkens back to our old friend Tommy Douglas and the introduction of universal medical coverage in Saskatchewan in 1962. The province's doctors were against the scheme, as we discussed earlier, considering Douglas's plan a threat to clinical decision-making and professional autonomy — especially when it came to billing patients and collecting their fees. Following the twenty-three-day Saskatchewan doctors' strike, a compromise was reached, known as the Saskatoon Agreement, that basically acknowledged doctors were independent contractors who'd be paid on a fee-for-service basis from that point on.

When medicare was eventually rolled out in the rest of Canada, starting in 1968, primary care continued to be delivered by physicians working in solo practices or in small groups where overhead and expenses could be shared. The focus was on providing basic medical services, with little thought about preventing illness or promoting wellness. After-hours care was pretty much non-existent, which resulted in patients having no choice but to visit hospital emergency departments after hours and on weekends — a pricey alternative that ate up a hell of a lot of health care resources unnecessarily. To make matters worse, the fee-for-service model also discouraged other health care providers from becoming involved in the delivery of primary care, as there was no practical way for a family doctor to reimburse them for their services.

Thanks in no small part to the heroic — and, frankly, often unappreciated efforts of primary care reform pioneers like Dr. Wendy Graham and others — things finally began to change around the turn of the century. As mentioned, the Harris government dipped its toe in the river of primary care reform and launched a series of pilot projects in 1999, which would be studied and measured against the current fee-for-service system. After Mike Harris stepped down as premier of Ontario in 2002, and his successor Ernie Eves failed to win re-election in 2003, the Liberals, led by Premier Dalton McGuinty and Health Minister George Smitherman, expanded the program and launched a number of their own primary care reform models — FHGs, FHNs, FHOs, FHTs (in plain English: family health groups, family health networks, family health organizations, and family health teams) — which soon became known as the aforementioned alphabet soup. It should be pointed out that one of the reasons the Ontario Liberals were able to so aggressively embrace primary care reform is because their federal cousins up in Ottawa provided a much-needed injection of new money through both the Primary Health Care Transition Fund and the Health Reform Fund, which targeted primary care, home care, and catastrophic drug coverage.

As a result of these rather dramatic changes to physician remuneration — although each was slightly different from the others, for the most part the new models relied on incentives and bonuses — more and more patients were suddenly able to find a family doctor and receive the kind of care they had previously only been able to dream of. Unfortunately — and this is where the law of unintended consequences once again rears its ugly head — focusing on prevention and wellness instead of simply treating sickness proved to be expensive. *Very* expensive. Between 2007 and 2009, for example, total payments to primary care doctors increased by 32 percent (compared to a 23 percent increase in overall health care expenditures by the Ontario government). This increase was largely a result of these new reimbursement models. During this same period, primary care health care expenditures rose from 7.5 to 8.1 percent of the health care budget, while payments to primary care physicians increased by 31 percent, compared to an increase of 25 percent for all Ontario physicians. Not surprisingly, this primary care physician "gravy train" had a great deal to do with reversing the trend of new graduates shunning primary care and becoming specialists instead, something that had been affecting the supply of family doctors and general practitioners since the early 1990s.

By 2012, Ontario was shovelling over $1 billion a year into primary care reform and had enrolled three-quarters of the province's population and three-quarters of the province's family doctors into one of these new models. Patients — read "voters" — loved being able to access their doctor, or at least a member of his or her team, after hours, as well as having the opportunity to take advantage of auxiliary services, such as dietitians and other health care professionals, all at the same convenient location. But while our elected officials were touting the benefits of the changes they'd made to the way the province delivered primary care, civil servants were warning their political masters the plan simply wasn't sustainable. For one thing, there seemed to be no obvious way of measuring outcomes. Did keeping Ontarians healthier, for instance, truly offset the cost of paying family doctors all this extra money instead of just paying them to deal with patients only when they got sick?

Needless to say, it would have been easier to monitor the costs and benefits of this new system if the government had had access to better data. This data was supposed to come from electronic medical records (EMR), which were meant to be an integral part of primary care reform. Remember, the main idea behind reforming primary care in the first place was to improve the patient experience by integrating different health care providers and having them look after patients all in one place, so it only made sense to have a system that could keep track of records, test results, and prescription renewals in a similar manner. Sadly, this was not to be, mainly as a result of the massive fumble (which I'll talk about in more detail in a few moments) that occurred when the province went down the electronic medical records path without a flashlight or a road map. Stupid is as stupid does, I believe someone once said. In the end, the EMR system created offered no benefits to patients — and no cost savings to the government.

And so it was that in 2008, in the midst of a global economic meltdown, Ontario found itself between a rock and a hard place. While the government wanted to continue to offer Ontarians — again, read "voters" — a Cadillac health care system, the reality was they could only afford to pay for a Volkswagen.

The province had arrived at a crossroads and was facing a huge dilemma. How could it continue to fund the new primary health care models that were proving to be so much more costly than the old ones when the economy had gone down the tubes? And what would the fallout be if the new models were changed or cancelled? Patients had overwhelmingly embraced them and the evidence would seem to suggest — albeit not definitively — that patient outcomes were improving. Good questions.

For Ontario Health Minister Eric Hoskins, the answer was simple. Hoskins, who, don't forget, was himself a doctor and surely knew better, decided the best way to deflect blame from the Liberal government's fiscal mismanagement was to vilify the province's doctors. After accusing a number of the province's highest billers of "ripping off" the province and greedily putting their needs ahead of those of their patients, the health minister then unilaterally decided to limit the number of family doctors entering alternative payment models. At the same time, Dr. Hoskins cut all fees by 2.65 percent, and refused to negotiate a new Physician Services Agreement with the Ontario Medical Association, even though the province's doctors had been without a contract for a number of years.

Interestingly enough, had the health minister simply taken the time to read the auditor general's report from 2011, which tried to make sense of the province's crazy quilt of seventeen — that's right, I said *seventeen* — different alternative payment plans, he'd have discovered for himself just how unpalatable providing primary care in Ontario had become. For example, the auditor general revealed, 22 percent of patients enrolled with doctors in the most popular alternative payment plans never paid their family doctor a visit in 2009–10. And yet, doctors took in something on the order of $123 million simply for having "rostered" these invisible patients. To make matters worse, nearly half of those patients saw another doctor that year — this was a big no-no and flew in the face of the spirit of the plan. These extra visits resulted in the Ontario Health Insurance Plan paying additional money to cover the costs of the services provided by the doctors outside the plans. The auditor general also discovered the vast majority of doctors who'd enrolled in these alternative payment plans were making on average at least 25 percent more than their counterparts who were still charging fee-for-service.

I can't help recalling, all these years later, a question I heard Premier Harris ask Dr. Graham about primary care reform somewhere back in the late 1990s. It was at one of those events where the room is filled with lobbyists and others with an agenda who will stop at nothing to get a moment of a cabinet minister's, or in this case the premier's, time. At any rate, Premier Harris leaned across me after I had introduced him to Dr. Graham, labelling her "the architect of primary care reform" — a silly remark, as the two often shared a plane from North Bay to Toronto on business and didn't need me to make any kind of introduction — and asked one simple question. "Will it work?"

I don't recall Dr. Graham's answer, as someone called my name and asked me to come over and introduce them to some other luminary, but she could easily have answered, "Yes and no." For, while the implementation of primary care reform in the province of Ontario was responsible for nearly 1.5 million Ontarians who'd been without a family doctor for years finally being able to secure one after joining that doctor's roster, the fact is, when you turn doctors into civil servants, they'll likely start acting like them. I mean, who wouldn't want to be paid for not seeing patients?

It's only human nature.

Electronic Medical Records

If information technology is all about making the complex *simple*, then surely the Ontario government's approach to creating an electronic medical records system for the province was all about making the simple *complex*. Fifteen years and $8 billion later, Ontario still doesn't have an eHealth system that works. How could this have happened? How could such a good idea have ended up costing so much money, only to end in failure? It almost seems unfathomable. And yet, that's just what happened in Ontario.

To understand why, it's first necessary to take a step back and examine why there was such a hunger to convert from paper records to electronic records in the first place. Having worked with doctors for many years, I had a front-row seat during the late 1990s and early 2000s when talk about e-medicine was just beginning to heat up. Although almost everyone agreed the current system was inefficient and potentially put patients at risk unnecessarily, few were anxious to undertake the daunting task of converting millions of pages of handwritten notes and test results to an electronic format.

The argument for making the change, though, was quite strong. By allowing doctors to search patient records quickly and efficiently, an electronic medical record, in theory, makes it possible for doctors to identify patients who're behind on their vaccinations or due for cancer-screening tests. With the click of a button, a patient can be notified without delay to book an appointment to take care of the problem before their next visit to the doctor. Electronic records can also be used as a patient education tool. For instance, with a couple of clicks, a doctor can create an electronic chart that monitors how well a diabetic patient's blood-sugar levels are being controlled. But the biggest advantage of going digital — and this was the major selling point I heard over and over again, both from doctors and hospital administrators — was that a linked system would allow the easy exchange of diagnostic results and other information between a patient's primary care provider and other health care practitioners. This alone would justify the high cost and inconvenience of converting to such a system, everyone said, because it would help patients receive care in a timelier fashion, while avoiding the costly duplication of tests — especially if that person arrived in the emergency department of their local hospital, unconscious or unable to speak.

Unfortunately, instead of working on finding a solution to this problem collegially, each province set about tackling the problem in a different way. Alberta set a goal back in 1997 of creating a single repository of health care information for everyone in the province. This included things like laboratory and radiology test results, hospitalization reports, and lists of prescriptions. True, the road to digitalization was not without its challenges — not the least of which was getting the province's doctors onside and dealing with the thorny issue of patient confidentiality and privacy — but Alberta pretty much accomplished its goal on time and on target in spite of everything. The province even opened up a secure online portal that permitted patients to review their own health data.

In Ontario, where the province made a bad strategic decision right from the get-go, opting for a local approach that collects data into regional hubs, it's been a different story. While the health ministry had hoped to eventually connect the various networks together, Ontario's auditor general found that by 2015 the province still hadn't met its own target of having a fully operational electronic medical record system operating in Ontario. As if that isn't bad enough, no one to this day knows for sure when patients in Ontario will be able to access their own medical records and test results via a portal the way Albertans can.

Now, to be fair, the challenge facing those charged with coming up with a viable, affordable, and efficient eHealth system in the province of Ontario was indeed formidable. Among other things, they had to digitally link roughly 30,000 doctors, 150,000 nurses, thousands of other health care providers, 238 hospitals, 36 public health units, 76 community health care centres, more than 4,000 pharmacies, 23 community laboratories and nearly 1,000 independent clinics.

After the government's first attempt ended in failure — Smart Systems for Health Agency, which wasted in excess of $650 million — Premier Dalton McGuinty brought in Dr. Alan Hudson to head up Ontario's new eHealth agency. Dr. Hudson, who had an impressive resumé and a solid track record when it came to fixing the unfixable, seemed at the time an inspired choice. One of the first things he did was hire Sarah Kramer as eHealth's chief executive officer. Kramer also had an extraordinary resumé and track record, having successfully brought the Province of Nova Scotia's health system into the digital age.

But then the law of unintended consequences reared its head in a most ugly and unexpected way. Because Sarah Kramer believed — rightly or wrongly — she had been hired by Dr. Hudson with the full support of Premier McGuinty, she decided to ignore the health ministry's normal procurement procedures. As a result, the ministry's eHealth branch, which had fewer than thirty full-time employees, soon employed an army of consultants — at one point, more than three hundred consultants were working on the project and billing incredible amounts of money. One consultant, for example, charged the Government of Ontario $2,700 per day. Another consultant, who billed $300 an hour, charged the government for reading an article on electronic medical records, which had been given to her by her husband, another consultant. Two other consultants, serving as vice-presidents, were regularly flown back and forth from their homes in Alberta. As if this wasn't bad enough, some of those same consultants had the gall to charge taxpayers $1.65 for a cup of tea and $3.99 for cookies.

Not surprisingly, heads eventually rolled. Following the release of a scathing report by the auditor general, Health Minister David Caplan resigned. CEO Sarah Kramer also stepped down, but not before receiving $317,000 in compensation for her ten months of "work" — this on top of the $114,000 bonus she received after having been hired in the first place. Sadly, Dr. Hudson became a casualty of this fiasco, as well, quietly resigning shortly after Ms. Kramer was forced to walk the plank. The departures came after the two opposition parties accused the McGuinty government of doling out over $5 million in untendered contracts to consultants, many of whom had links to the Liberals. Documents released by the government a few months later, as a result of a number of freedom of information requests, show that the number was closer to $16 million.

Granted, every government in Canada — whether we're talking federal, provincial, territorial, or municipal — uses consultants. They tend to bring specific skill sets to the table to complete well-defined tasks that are often beyond the capabilities of government employees. Elected officials like having the option of using consultants because they find it easier to convince the public they're not increasing the size of the bureaucracy — to mention nothing of the "independent" nature of their advice, which can either be taken or ignored, depending upon which way the political winds are blowing. And, of course, I'd be remiss in not reminding you that I, too, have worked as a consultant, billing clients $250 an hour or $5,000 to $10,000 a month for my services. But the problem with what happened in Ontario is that all these years and billions of dollars later, we still don't appear to have any hope of finding our way through the digital maze that is electronic medical records. Had all these consultants managed to come up with an eHealth system that actually worked, I guarantee you we wouldn't be talking about how much it cost or shaking our heads at the gall of someone making hundreds of dollars an hour charging us for refreshments. For one of the truisms of politics is that no one remembers who caused the problem. They only remember who fixed it — even if the one who fixes the problem was the same person or group who created the problem in the first place. Regrettably, for the Ontario Liberals, their failure to find a solution to the province's eHealth problem was yet another of the many reasons Ontario voters kicked them to the curb on June 7, 2018.

The Transformation Agenda

The Chinese have a saying — a curse, actually: "May you live in interesting times." Now, some have claimed there never was such a saying, that the aforementioned "curse" is in reality a bastardization of the following ancient Chinese idiom: "It's better to be a dog in a peaceful time than be a man in a chaotic period." Either way, I'm sure you'll agree with me that the times we're currently living in — some would say, "suffering through" — are, if nothing else, truly interesting. The Ontario Liberal government's Transformation Agenda, which helped usher in a "reign of error" that lasted fifteen years, was particularly responsible for making these times noteworthy. So, without further ado, here are a couple of examples that illustrate rather nicely what happens when ideology gets in the way of common sense, when know-it-all politicians truly know nothing at all.

Read 'em and weep.

Exhibit A

The media release said it all. "Given the recent political developments in Ontario and uncertainty regarding timing relating thereto, the parties have agreed not to continue with the currently contemplated transaction." It was Friday, November 2, 2012. That was the day the deal died. The day Centric

Health announced it was terminating its proposed acquisition of Shouldice Hospital. That was the day we saw the first casualty of the Ontario Liberals so-called Transformation Agenda.

Many Canadians are familiar with the Shouldice name. Founded in 1945 by Dr. Edward Earle Shouldice, this private, for-profit hospital has been offering the finest in hernia care not only to Canadians but to patients from all over the globe. "Grandfathered" in 1973 under a special provision in the Private Hospitals Act, Shouldice has continued to operate at its Thornhill, Ontario, location with one foot inside the Ontario health care system and one foot outside. Going there for hernia surgery is so commonplace that even the socialists' socialist, former federal NDP leader Jack Layton, chose Shouldice for his hernia surgery.

But all that changed on September 7, 2012. That was the date Centric Health put out a media release, announcing it had purchased the Shouldice Hospital for $14.5 million. Judging from the reaction of the usual suspects — Dr. Danielle Martin and the Canadian Doctors for Medicare group; Doris Grinspun and the Registered Nurses' Association; and other assorted naysayers and doomsday prophets — the world was about to come to an end. All because Dr. Jack Shevel, a South African doctor living in San Diego, California, had the audacity to try to add a true Canadian health care success story to his already impressive stable of partners.

The attacks on Dr. Shevel and Centric were as unfair as they were predictable. I'm paraphrasing but the gist of the argument went something like this: "How can we just stand by and let the Americans crash through the gates and pluck one of the jewels of our Canadian health care system right out from under us — especially after they've already had the cheek to grab up other Canadian health care winners like Blue Water Surgical Centre and Lifemark Health? Clearly, the time has come to take a stand and urge Deb Matthews to reject the sale and bring Shouldice fully back into the Ontario health care system family."

Under the provisions of the aforementioned Private Hospitals Act, the health minister does indeed have the right to accept or reject any sale of an enterprise such as Shouldice. Ironically, though, when Centric bought another private, for-profit hospital in Ontario a few years back — this would be the Don Mills Surgical Unit — there didn't seem to be nearly the outcry. Maybe that's because the company making the purchase then was the Canadian-owned Allegro Health Corporation, which later was bought up by Centric. But now that the big, bad American barbarians were at the gate … well, something had to be done.

This was truly a shame because the folks at Centric Health are all first-rate people — innovative entrepreneurs, who, while definitely interested in creating value for their shareholders, weren't looking to gut our health care system and destroy a gem like Shouldice. They merely wanted to bring the hernia facility under the Centric umbrella and continue to have it operate as a private hospital where most procedures would still be covered by public funding.

Of course, all that is off the table now. As for Shouldice, like a bride jilted at the altar by her groom, it was left in the unenviable position of having to find a new suitor. Sadly for Shouldice, suitors like Centric are few and far between.

Exhibit B

Having worked at Queen's Park once upon a time, I understand only too well that there's a huge amount of paperwork the average MPP has to dig through just to keep on top of issues and current events. To say nothing of what a minister of the Crown must digest every day in order to prepare for the daily grind of question period and media scrums. Unfortunately, there are times when our elected officials make mistakes, misinterpret data, or even deliberately mislead the public by misrepresenting the facts in order to score cheap political points. Such was the case with Canadian Plasma Resources.

Health Minister Deb Matthews climbed up on her high horse to portray herself as the defender of our Canadian blood services system, and brought forth a piece of legislation, the Voluntary Blood Donations Act, designed to ban pay-for-plasma, which effectively put one company, Canadian Plasma Resources, out of business — this after they had invested over seven million dollars in three Ontario clinics in hopes of creating 150 highly paid, skilled jobs.

Not surprisingly, the minister enlisted the help of not one but two medical ethicists — Margaret Somerville, the founding director of the McGill Centre for Medicine, Ethics and Law, and Lisa Schwartz, a health care ethicist from McMaster University — to convince the public she was right to take the stance she did.

"You have to look at what value is upheld by the fact we give our blood," Ms. Somerville said. "That is the value of altruism. When you make that an economic relationship, you corrupt that value. It takes away from the value of the gift, even if some people continue to give their blood."

"You worry about going down that slippery slope toward the sale of organs and the sale of embryos," Ms. Schwartz said. "We need to keep a tight rein on this."

"You've got this further worry about the exploitation of poor people, who don't have any other options and who are desperate for money," Ms. Somerville added.

Dr. Barzin Bahardoust, Canadian Plasma Resources chief executive officer, responded in the following way:

> Ontario's need for lifesaving drugs made from human plasma far exceeds our ability to produce it. That's why Ontario's health care system purchases hundreds of millions of dollars of these products from American companies that compensate plasma donors. No country in the world is self-sufficient in the production of these products from a solely voluntary donor base. This is not about collecting blood or plasma for transfusion, but rather plasma that will be manufactured into critical pharmaceutical products for patients with life-threatening diseases.

Matthews' hypocrisy on this one was especially infuriating. While she was quick to take a position that paying people for their time so they can donate their plasma somehow takes advantage of the disadvantaged in Ontario, she apparently had no problem with exploiting the poor in the United States in order to ensure there'd be enough plasma to meet Canada's needs.

Even the Canadian Hemophilia Society agreed with Canadian Plasma Resources that the minister of health was just plain wrong to ban pay-for-plasma, issuing a statement that said, in part: "The decision by the Government of Ontario not to allow these centres to open is a reaction to public opinion, not a decision based on science or ethics. Over the last twenty years, the plasma industry has developed well-documented and effective procedures to ensure that plasma can be collected safely, both for donors and the recipients."

Canadian Plasma Resources was not out to exploit the poor or to put our blood supply at risk. Of course the company wanted to make a profit, but it also wanted to bring innovation and jobs to Ontario. Far from being a threat to the people of Ontario, it was trying to do something truly heroic. If only our boneheaded elected officials had had the good sense to get the hell out of the way. How do I know this? Because, unlike Deb Matthews, I actually went to the trouble of meeting with Dr. Bahardoust at one of his clinics in downtown Toronto to find out for myself what was fact and what was fiction when it comes to paying for plasma.

Here's what I discovered:

Fact: Currently, only three of the roughly thirty plasma-derived therapies used by Canadians are manufactured, in part, from plasma collected from unpaid donors by Canadian Blood Services and Héma-Québec. The rest all come from paid U.S. donors.

Fact: Because Canada requires 1,100,000 litres of plasma per annum to meet the demand in this country, the only way to ensure sufficient access to that supply is through giving incentives to donors, to encourage repeat donations.

Fact: If allowed to institute its pay-for-plasma system, Canadian Plasma Resources would be able to produce as much as 400,000 litres of plasma per annum by 2020, which would increase the level of Canadian self-sufficiency to nearly half of what's needed.

Fact: The company planned to invest a further $300 million and build Canada's first-ever plasma refractory, which would create another three thousand jobs and go a long way toward securing our country's plasma supply.

Not surprisingly, this story didn't have a happy ending. Thanks to Deb Matthews and the Liberals' Transformation Agenda, Canadian Plasma Resources was chased away, taking its money, jobs, and investments with it.

The most frightening words you'll ever hear? Simple. "I'm from the government and I'm here to help."

Choosing Wisely

On the surface, Choosing Wisely, a Canadian-based health education campaign that was launched in the spring of 2014, seemed like a good idea. The brainchild of University of Toronto professor Dr. Wendy Levinson, in conjunction with the Canadian Medical Association, the campaign was meant to assist doctors and patients to engage in a meaningful dialogue about unnecessary tests, treatments, and procedures, so they could make informed choices that would not only save our health care system money but also result in better, more positive outcomes for the patient. The thinking here was that unnecessary interventions by physicians often do more harm than good, by exposing patients to needless risks and potentially the stress and anxiety of having to undergo even more tests to investigate so-called false positive test results. By forcing doctors to stop and reconsider how they have traditionally practised medicine, those behind the Choosing Wisely campaign hoped physicians would be more inclined to lean on the most recent evidence when deciding on the best course of action for treating individual patients. Equally important, the campaign would serve as an educational tool for patients, who often feel that "more care is better care," even though the evidence doesn't bear this out.

At the core of the Choosing Wisely campaign is a list of things that doctors and patients should question. This list includes things such as specific tests, treatments, or procedures commonly chosen by doctors but which are either not evidence-based or could expose patients to unnecessary risks. For instance, one of Dr. Levinson's first recommendations was "Don't order screening chest X-rays and ECGs for asymptomatic or low risk outpatients." Other recommendations soon followed, based upon the following criteria: the development process behind each recommendation must be thoroughly documented and publicly available; each recommendation must be within the recommending specialty's scope of practice; the tests, treatments, or procedures included are to be those that are frequently used, and that may expose patients to harm or stress; and each recommendation must be supported by evidence.

Like a brush fire, the Choosing Wisely campaign began to spread. Health care stakeholder groups in Alberta, Atlantic Canada, Ontario, and Quebec were established to help convince provincial governments to embrace the concept of choosing wisely. At the local level, hospitals, regional health authorities, and medical associations tried to find innovative ways of putting the campaign's recommendations into practice. Even Canada's medical schools got into the act, introducing new content into the curriculum that would challenge students to stop and think and make decisions differently than they might otherwise have done. Those responsible for the Choosing Wisely campaign also built important relationships with patient groups and media outlets in hopes of developing and disseminating material meant to increase patient awareness, as well as supporting them in conversations with their doctor about appropriate levels of care. A bilingual mobile app, available on both Android and Apple platforms, containing all physician recommendations and patient educational materials was also developed.

There is a problem with the Choose Wisely program, however: all of the risk and all of the costs are borne by doctors.

Forcing Canada's physicians to "choose wisely" results in them having to make choices that can result in their personal risk increasing dramatically. Remember, we live in a litigious age. As a result, doctors often feel they have no choice but to practise what they call "defensive medicine." This means they'll order more tests than necessary, or have patients undergo questionable procedures, simply as a way of protecting their backsides. And really, who can blame them? Thanks in no small part to the internet and Dr. Google, patients are now armed with more information (both accurate and inaccurate) than ever before. It's not unusual to see a patient or their family members demand an MRI or a CT scan — even if there's little clinical evidence for ordering one.

If doctors don't order such tests or prescribe drugs, whether necessary or not, not only do they risk getting sued, they also face a loss of income. Unless a physician is part of a group practice, where they are paid an annual lump sum for seeing patients on their roster instead of being paid fee-for-service, they might be significantly affecting their bottom line by practising conservative medicine. Remember, many doctors — particularly specialists such as cardiologists — have set up clinics where patients can go for tests without having to wait weeks and weeks for the results. These clinics and all that expensive machinery are paid for out of the doctors' own pockets. The government, for its part, pays only a small fee for the conducting of the test. By forcing doctors to reduce the number of tests they order, we might well be cutting off our nose to spite our face. After all, pretty much every doctor is running a small business — employing staff, paying taxes, and offering an important service to the community. Medicine is not a charity. If you make it impossible to make a profit — even a small one — you risk putting that doctor out of business, which ultimately will have a huge impact on patient care.

Instead of choosing wisely, a better idea might be for the government to either properly fund our health care system or — if they can't or won't — then free it. As I've said elsewhere, Canadians should have every right to make our own health care decisions — especially when it comes to deciding what we want to spend our health care dollars on. Putting our doctors into the unsavoury position of having to *ration* health care is, in my opinion, neither wise nor much of a choice.

— PART IV —

THE BIG FIX

So, what's wrong with our health care system? The problem, to my way of thinking, is threefold.

First, when those in charge first started pondering how they might change the way health care was delivered, back in the late 1950s and early 1960s, much of what they came up with was ideologically driven. Or, to put it another way, borrowing modern medical lingo, it wasn't evidence-based. As is often the case when politics rears its ugly head, the process for creating good public policy can be hijacked by those with their own agenda, people who'll stop at nothing to get their way. One of their tricks — straight out of the old spin-doctor handbook, I'm afraid — is to substitute *emotion* for *logic*. In other words, they try to get decision-makers to think with their *hearts* instead of their *heads*. This is what I believe happened when today's health care system was being conceived.

To make matters worse, no one involved in the original exercise — be it politicians, civil servants, or those leading the charge for the introduction of a publicly funded health care system — seemed to be looking far enough ahead into the future.

The second problem — and it's a big one — is that our health care system isn't really a "system" at all. As I pointed out earlier, it's an insurance scheme, and a badly run one at that. I mean, stop and think about it for a moment. How can we call it a health care system when so many things aren't covered? Like eyes, for instance. Or teeth. And don't get me started on the bean-counters, with their infuriating and frequently incoherent and inconsistent rules regarding what medicare covers and what it doesn't. Furthermore, what kind of a system would allow patients — including some of our sickest and most vulnerable citizens, often seniors — to clog up the hallways of hospital emergency departments, all because our long-term care facilities are unable to accommodate them? "Bed-blockers," hospital administrators call them. "Human beings," I call them.

The third problem with our health care system is a little harder to explain, but pretty much comes down to the fact that the Canada Health Act features five main principles: public administration, comprehensiveness, universality, portability, and accessibility. Notice what's missing? *Quality*. Nowhere do we measure, offer, or even seem to care about making sure that quality is part of our health care system here in Canada. Unlike the Ford Motor Company, whose famous commercial from the 1980s — "At Ford, Quality is Job One" — touted the importance of caring about the quality of one's work, those responsible for medicare decided long ago that quality, at least when it comes to health care, is a frill, something we can all live without.

Except, of course, we can't. Because if quality doesn't matter, then neither do outcomes. Which means that whether we survive an encounter with our health care system or not is irrelevant. A life lost is the same as a life saved — at least as far as the civil service is concerned — simply because the line gets shorter. This is why, when we're talking about properly diagnosing illnesses, ensuring patients receive treatment in a timely manner, and ultimately saving lives, one can't help feeling that when it comes to medicare in Canada, "Quality is Job None."

By now, you might well be asking yourself, "What qualifies you to comment on the failings of our health care system, and why should we believe your prescription for reforming medicare is any better than anyone else's?"

I guess my response to that would go something like this: In the same way it takes a thief to catch a thief, in order to cut through all the lies and

BS coming out of the mouths of our elected officials and defenders of the status quo when it comes to health care, you need someone who understands the difference between something being *true* and something being *believable*. Though the difference is subtle — and is difficult to spot at times — it can be detected, so long as you speak the language and know how to listen carefully.

Politicians are a lot like Pinocchio, as I'm sure everyone is aware of by now. They use weasel words and phrases like, "It's not our intention …" or "We have no plans at this time …" or "To be perfectly honest …" They talk about "making investments," and "being transparent," and go to great lengths to tell us poor dumb Canadians why it's important to stand up and be defenders of that which makes us different from our neighbours to the south. Typically, when they say things like that they're talking about our health care system. It's all hogwash, of course, but it makes for good sound bites.

The sad truth is that when it comes to politics, perception is more important than reality. In fact, some have gone even further, saying that perception *is* reality. Think about that for a moment. Perception is reality. Taken to its extreme, this philosophy argues that so long as what's coming out of someone's mouth is *believable*, then it must be, for all intents and purposes, the *truth* — even if it isn't. This probably explains why so many of our leaders are nothing more than a bevy of blathering buffoons — talking heads who look good, sound good, and seem to make sense, all while talking nonsense.

Obviously, we need to talk. By way of kick-starting the conversation, let me offer a little free advice. Although we all know what that's worth, you really should listen to me, since I've spent most of the past twenty-five years in the trenches — if not exactly fighting side by side with doctors and nurses and other health care providers, then at least as a passionate observer. Think of me as a war correspondent, if you will, or perhaps a "canary in the coal mine."

And just what have I witnessed during this time? One bad decision after another, made by one politician after another, over and over and over again. Things are indeed a bloody mess when it comes to health care — and it's about to get worse.

But there is hope.

Here are ten things we could do tomorrow to reinvent and ultimately fix Canada's health care system. By no means are these the only changes we need to consider making to save medicare from a fate worse than death, but they represent a good start. And while I acknowledge many of my recommendations might be somewhat controversial, doing nothing is *not* an option. We've already wasted too much time pretending everything's all right. The health care doomsday clock is ticking. We don't have the luxury of putting this off any longer.

1. Stop Lying to Us

Politicians tell lies all the time. They lie by omission. They lie by commission. They mislead the public, often by releasing reports chock full of irrelevant information and statistics. They engage in misdirection, usually by making an announcement of some sort, which inevitably turns into a photo op, typically involving large sums of taxpayer dollars being doled out like candy at Halloween, to distract the public from the issue at hand or some crisis. They give names to pieces of legislation that mean the opposite to what the bill actually entails. They exaggerate, they fabricate, and they minimize.

Even worse, they say things like: "We're transforming our health care system." Into what? I have no idea. They tell us: "We all have to choose wisely — especially doctors — in order to make sure we spend our limited health care dollars as intelligently as possible."

This is all well and good but … we'd be wise to keep in mind that in 1964, the year Justice Emmett Hall issued his initial report on the state of health care here in Canada, health care expenditures in this country totalled $3 billion. Fifty-five years later, that amount has ballooned to over $200 billion — give or take a few million. Anyone who thinks that's sustainable, or in any way affordable, is either delusional or a liar.

Or both.

How Might We?

To understand why our elected officials are so addicted to telling lies, we must first take a look at the kinds of personality traits someone who runs for public office exhibits, as well as the myriad of reasons people decide to put their name forward to be a candidate in the first place. Whether you believe it or not, it takes a lot of courage to let your name stand on the ballot and put up with both the physical and the mental stress that come with the territory.

After all, should you be lucky enough to beat the odds and actually win a seat in the legislature, chances are that before you call it a day — four, eight, or maybe twelve years later — you'll likely have ruined your health, destroyed your marriage, and screwed up your kids for life. Think I'm kidding? The political landscape is littered with hundreds of politicos who've suffered nervous breakdowns, found themselves battling depression, and who've even, in some cases, committed suicide. To make matters worse, they often find themselves away from home for days — and, sometimes, weeks — at a time, leaving their spouses and children to fend for themselves.

Although every candidate is unique, most display the following attributes: they have a strong drive and plenty of ambition, they exhibit physical and mental toughness, and they have an ability to "see the big picture" and "get things done." As for why people decide to enter the political arena in the first place … well, the reasons are as unique as each candidate. Some do it because they want to make a difference. Others step up because they feel it's time for a change of government. Some want action on a specific issue. A few wish to give back to their community while others feel it's time to give *real* people a *real* voice. Then there are those who're keen to introduce innovative ideas. The ones who think it's possible to "do politics differently," or run government like a business. Finally, some are just plain curious to see if they're up to the challenge — they want to know if they can pull it off.

The most important thing to remember about a politician, however, is that from the moment they're elected right up until the time of the next election, they're constantly aware that whatever they do or say and whatever decisions they make will have an impact on their chances for re-election. Failure to understand this basic truth means you'll be destined not to succeed in your dealings with them. Trust me on this. I've been working with politicians for almost thirty years now. I've met with them one on one, face to face. I've appeared before them at legislative committees. I've had breakfast, lunch, and dinner with them. We've even enjoyed late-night cocktails together, back when I was still known to imbibe after hours. Like a scientist working in a strange and wonderful laboratory, I've learned a thing or two about how they think, feel, and act. First and foremost, they're not bad people. They just do bad things. Secondly, they're motivated by one thing and one thing only — fear. They're afraid of losing. They're afraid of being humiliated. They're afraid of being wrong. Hell, sometimes they're even afraid of showing they're afraid.

If we're to have any chance of getting our elected officials to stop lying to us, then we're going to have to convince them they don't have to be so afraid. And how do we do this? Well, to be frank, *we* have to quit lying to them ourselves. Instead, we have to be honest about what kind of government we want and how we want to be governed. When we're talking about health care, for instance, we need to let our leaders know, in no uncertain terms, that we understand our health care system, as it's currently configured, is *not* sustainable, and that the status quo is *not* an option. Most important of all, we simply must make it crystal clear to all of them that being honest with us about why we need to embrace the hybrid solution *now* — before it's too late — won't get them turfed out of office. In fact, if anything, we'll be more likely to support someone who's courageous enough to speak the truth for a change.

Why Would We Want To?

One of my main goals in writing this book has been to inject a little honesty into the debate. Whether searching the internet for news items about our crumbling health care system, monitoring social media via Facebook and Twitter, or listening to a seemingly endless number of talking heads debate the issues in whatever public forum they happen to be in, I've been nothing less than appalled by the number of nose-stretchers, if not out-and-out lies, people have been spewing about the state of things.

Year after year, health ministers all across the land have risen in their legislatures to report on the state of our health care union. No matter which party has been in power, at what level of government — federal, provincial, or territorial — those responsible for keeping us healthy and out of hospital have unfurled a carpet of lies, untruths, and fantasies of the most remarkable kind. A story about unicorns and rainbows might be appropriate when you're writing a children's book. But when you're talking about health care, this just won't do.

What's missing, to my way of thinking — and what we so desperately need — is a *plan*. And not just a one- or two-year plan. No, no, no. We need a ten-year plan. Those of us who use and rely on our health care system need to know it'll be there for us when we need it — today, tomorrow, and well into the future.

Medicare, as it's currently structured, will likely implode sometime within the next decade, collapsing under the strain put on it by our growing and aging population and the high cost of all these new drugs, technologies, and treatments — to mention nothing of the looming doctor shortage, the result of our aging and extremely pissed-off medical professionals deciding to either retire early or leave Canada altogether in search of greener pastures. Oh, and did I mention those three tsunamis that are brewing and bubbling out there, just on the horizon, waiting to swamp us and flood the boat? Obesity, diabetes, and dementia? I think I might have. If you're looking for something to be afraid of, these three will do quite nicely, thank you very much. This is why it's so important we come up with a ten-year plan right now — *today* — to figure out how we're going to deal with all this stuff. Unfortunately, as pretty much every politician will tell you, they don't have ten years — they only have four years, at best, before they'll have to face the electorate again.

This is where we come in. We have to let them know we'll give them the necessary time to get it right, that we understand Rome wasn't built in a day, and that reinventing our country's health care system is going to take a whole lot of time and a great deal of patience. If some leader, some party, develops a workable, sensible plan that will get us back on track by committing to the major restructuring our health care system needs, then we — the voters — *have* to band together and throw our support behind those people to help them form a government. I mean, let's face it. Medicare is such a mess because we keep turfing our governments — changing them as often as a baby's diapers, or so it seems. As we have seen, all this "toing and froing," all this "left-ing and then right-ing" is what's killing us … literally. If we're to have any hope of fixing what's wrong with our health care system, then we need to pick a plan, get behind the plan, and stick with the plan. Lurching from one bad idea to another is no way to operate. We need some serious stability to create an environment where outside-the-box thinking is not only encouraged but embraced. So long as the status quo is a "no go," the future will indeed be bright. But only if we have the courage to be honest with each other.

What's Stopping Us from Doing So?

While it might be easy to blame government for the crisis we're facing, I say it's wrong for us to go down that road. There's plenty of blame to go around. We're all guilty here. We've all been part of the problem and we can all be part of the solution. But first, we have to admit there actually *is* a problem. Since medicare was introduced in Canada back in 1968, everyone seems to have been playing some sort of weird game called Let's Pretend. The reality is our country no longer has the best health care system in the world — not even close. Nor is there enough money to keep medicare from collapsing under its own weight. To put it plainly: our health care credit card is way over its limit and the payment is due.

Before we go any further, though, let me just say something shocking.

Although politicians have caused us an incredible amount of grief with their lies and deceit, the bigger problem, as far as I'm concerned, is the role Canada's doctors, nurses, and other health care professionals have played in the demise of our health care system. By propping up medicare, by going the extra mile and sticking their collective fingers into every hole the dike has sprung, our health care heroes have, in reality, made things way worse. For, you see, if they'd only sat back and let things fall apart the way any sensible person would, then they'd have forced the hands of our elected officials, leaving them no choice but to do something about all this years ago. Regrettably, doctors and nurses don't think that way. No matter how bad the conditions they're working under, no matter how lacking they are in resources, there's something in their nature that demands they persevere — no matter the consequences.

The other culprits when it comes to perpetrating the Big Lie, not surprisingly, are the unions. Whether we're talking nurses, or other health care providers, those who're unionized feel threatened by the likes of Dr. Brian Day and others who are pushing so hard for the hybrid solution because they're afraid of a little competition and worried that the introduction of a parallel private health care system may well have a detrimental effect on their wages and benefits. Now, I personally don't have any problems with unions. I consider former CAW president Buzz Hargrove a friend and count him as one of my most important mentors. I've also run job actions for various police unions during my long and varied career as a consultant. But the fact remains unions aren't being helpful when it comes to our country's ongoing health care debate.

However, the biggest impediment to the truth is us — we, the people — each and every citizen of this great country. Judging by the way we keep voting in bad and deceitful governments, we're, without a doubt, addicted to the candy they keep bribing us with. You can see it every time an election rolls around. They open up their wallets, they unlock the vaults, they start throwing money out the window ... showering voters with pre-election goodies, designed to fool us into believing they have our best interests at heart. If things are ever going to change, *we* must change. We have to stop letting candidates dupe us so easily. We especially have to stop them from getting away with not talking about the most important issue of all — health care — during the four or five weeks of the actual election campaign like they always seem to do. No, instead of pretending everything is fine, that there's nothing to see here, isn't it about high time we had a serious discussion about the future of medicare? After all, as someone once said, "If you don't stand for something, you'll fall for anything."

2. Put Patients First, Ideology Second

Like the *Titanic*, our health care system is about to hit a gigantic iceberg and will sink — sooner rather than later — mainly because those in charge keep putting ideology ahead of patient care. In Ontario, for instance, former health minister George Smitherman was given the task by Premier Dalton McGuinty of turning our health care system on its head and coming up with something new. Hence the birth of the Transformation Agenda. When that didn't work, Deb Matthews was brought in to get costs under control and bring "transparency" to the Ministry of Health and Long-Term Care. A few years later, it was Dr. Eric Hoskins's turn to try to make a silk purse out of a sow's ear. None of these "solutions" actually solved the problem. That's because they were designed to fix *political* problems, not the problems patients have. It kind of reminds me of the city planner who once said of Toronto's subway system, "If only the trains didn't have any passengers, there'd never be any delays to service."

This pretty much sums up what's wrong with all these schemes and dreams. The inconvenient truth is that our health care system is full to bursting with real, live, actual patients. And while buzzwords like "transformation" and "transparency" sound good in a fifteen-second clip on TV or radio, the reality is health care is a complicated, costly enterprise that's quickly threatening to eat up every last dollar available to government. We simply can't afford to continue down this road, pretending everything will turn out all right if only the bean-counters can figure out what to do about all those pesky patients, who keep turning up in doctors' offices or emergency departments, wanting someone to look after them.

How Might We?

When I was a young boy, growing up in the 1960s, governments at all three levels — federal, provincial, and municipal — were a force for good. They built things — highways, hospitals, and universities. They invested in our future and were led by people who worked hard to make life better for everyone, no matter their lot in life. Clearly, Canada's political leaders were dedicated to improving the lives of our country's citizens.

John Robarts, the premier of Ontario from 1961 to 1971, was just such a leader. Fuelled by a robust economy and aided by a talented group of cabinet ministers — including future Ontario premier and nation builder Bill Davis, who was Robarts's education minister for much of the decade before taking over as premier in 1971 — John Robarts made sure shovels not only went into the ground but that money went into our pockets. His list of accomplishments is as long as it is impressive. GO Transit. Ontario Place. The Ontario Science Centre. The province's first nuclear plant. A brand spanking new community college system, along with a number of modern universities, including Brock, Lakehead, Trent, and York. All this in addition to providing more funding for the Catholic school system, creating the Niagara Escarpment Commission, and bringing medicare to Ontario. Times were good, people looked forward to a bright future, and government was seen not so much as a necessary evil, but more like an entity that did things *for* people.

Fast-forward to today. More and more, we find ourselves living in a "Nanny State." Reminiscent of the old 1950s TV show *Father Knows Best*, left-leaning governments — and here I'm thinking of the Ontario Liberals under Dalton McGuinty and Kathleen Wynne; the NDP in Alberta and British Columbia; and the federal Liberals up in Ottawa — continually introduce legislation and bring in programs designed not to make our lives better or easier but, instead, with an eye toward influencing our behaviour. "Social engineering," it's called. As a result, in 2019, government is no longer seen as an entity that does things for people. Now, it does things *to* people.

Let's take the issue of raising the minimum wage, for example. Now, no one can argue against the need to help those who, through no fault of their own, find themselves at the bottom of the socio-economic scale. And while we may not need to go as far as playing the role of our brother's keeper, I think we can all agree it's good for society as a whole if those of us who're doing a little better offer our fellow citizens a "hand up" instead of a "handout." But when Kathleen Wynne decided to increase the minimum wage in Ontario from $11.60 an hour to $14.00 an hour all in one fell swoop, it's no wonder all hell broke loose. Companies, unable to absorb the extra $6,000 per year per full-time employee, were left with no choice but to try to figure out creative ways to offset these added costs. Some decided to do away with paid breaks. Others cut employee benefits or increased the waiting period for those benefits to kick in. Still others told their employees they were no longer allowed to pocket tips but had to put the money into the till at the end of their shift. As if this wasn't bad enough, hundreds of workers lost their jobs, as a result of "mom-and-pop" shops shutting down operations or, in some cases, declaring bankruptcy.

Talk about the law of unintended consequences. As one Tim Hortons employee said, "I never asked for any of this. I was happy just having a job."

But changes to the province's labour laws were mild in comparison to the craziness Ontario's health minister, Dr. Eric Hoskins, introduced to the province's health care system at roughly the same time. In a seemingly endless effort to get it wrong and do as much damage as possible, Dr. Hoskins introduced a piece of legislation — the ironically named Patients First Act — that dramatically increased the number of civil servants managing the system, as well as allowing those same nameless, faceless officials to enter a physician's office, seize patient files, and generally upset the day-to-day operation of any clinic anywhere in Ontario.

Still, these things pale when placed side by side with Dr. Hoskins's pièce de résistance, the Protecting Patients Act, a bill I facetiously rechristened the You Can Look but You Better Not Touch Act. In this particular piece of legislation, the health minister — reacting in his own ham-handed way to a series of media reports, mostly by the *Toronto Star*, on sexual abuse by doctors — made it illegal for physicians to actually touch patients while examining them. Vaginal exams, rectal exams, breast exams. Doctors apparently could no longer be trusted to carry out these basic, life-saving investigations without a chaperone present — hired at the doctor's own expense, of course.

Perhaps someday someone will conduct a study into how many Ontario patients died as a result of Dr. Hoskins forcing physicians to practise "touchless medicine."

• • •

So, what can be done to make things better, to actually put patients first? Here are a few suggestions:

- Allow patients to choose where and from whom they wish to receive medical treatment.
- Allow doctors to deal directly with patients, rather than forcing physicians to be constantly weighed down by the swollen bureaucracies of provincial and territorial health ministries.
- Allow health care entities working outside of the government-sanctioned system more opportunity to provide services to patients.
- Reduce the number of health care civil servants, cutting any position that doesn't in some way directly support frontline care.
- Redirect the money saved from the elimination of these unnecessary positions so we can better fund basic health services.
- Give doctors the power to plan and assist with implementing the changes needed to improve Canada's health care system.

There is, of course, much more that could be done. But instituting these changes would go a long way toward making sure patients truly do come first.

Why Would We Want To?

Ensuring patients are the primary focus of our health care system will result in better quality care for all. Unfortunately, the way things work now, quality seemingly matters not one iota, and patients are all too often seen not as people, but rather as bed-blockers or numbers on wait-lists. We need to change our way of thinking about all this. We must move from focusing our efforts on trying to protect the status quo to doing everything possible to ensure patients receive the highest quality health care possible.

Needless to say, this will require a huge change in attitude. It will also require a major rethink as to where and how our health care dollars are spent. Currently, money is allocated by the federal government to the provinces, who then, in turn, give money to hospitals in either "blocks" or "envelopes" of funding. Doctors are typically paid fee-for-service — or, more and more, a kind of salary through a "capitation system" or a "blended payment" as part of a group practice, made up of other health care professionals such as nurse practitioners and nutritionists. Then there's a whole smorgasbord of other programs, featuring *targeted* funding — money meant to reduce wait times for hips and knees and cataracts, in hopes of buying votes from special interest groups.

What would make a lot more sense — at least, to my way of thinking — is if, instead of having the patient follow the funding, the funding were to follow the patient. This is referred to as "patient-centred care," and it's an idea whose time has come. If our goal is not just to treat the disease, but also to care for the entire patient — *holistically* — then the way medicare is currently set up is all wrong.

To use the car and mechanic metaphor ... medicine as it's practised here in Canada in the twenty-first century is a lot like the automobile repair business: someone waits until their car breaks down, then has it towed to their local garage, where they try with varying degrees of success to explain to the mechanic what the problem seems to be.

"It's making a funny noise," they'll tell the mechanic, in much the same way you or I might tell whoever's on call in the emergency department that evening, "I've got a mysterious pain ... right here." Both the doctor and the mechanic will then hook you or your car up to a machine and run a battery of tests in hopes of eliminating what could be wrong in order to figure out what actually is the problem.

Nothing wrong with that, I hear you say. So long as it works. Well, while it's true the way we deal with health care breakdowns might be fine in an emergency situation, there are problems having a system set up to function like this in non-emergency situations. Let me explain.

If your car is having trouble, you can have it looked at by any mechanic you like. Regrettably, this is not the case if you are experiencing issues with your health. Canada's health care system severely restricts your options when seeking out care. You may end up having to wait a long time see someone — whether it's for an appointment with your family doctor or to see a specialist. Because the health care system is currently designed to fund hospitals and doctors — not patients — people in need of care are forced to align their health care needs with our state-sanctioned and -funded system. That's because the ideology that would have us believe medicare is sacrosanct puts the system first, patients second.

If we had a patient-centred health care system, though, one whose principal goal was to provide quality medical care to patients, funding would follow individuals and they would have the freedom to spend any health care dollars allotted to them wherever they want. And if they wanted to spend more to obtain additional services, they could.

Isn't this the kind of two-tiered health care system the United States has? I hear you ask.

No, it isn't. Medicare would still exist, but it would exist in a much altered form. Patients would still have the money to cover their medical expenses, but they'd have greater freedom in choosing their doctors and hospitals. Hospitals would still receive basic funding, but both they and doctors would need to compete for patients' health care dollars by providing quality care. And if patients wanted to seek health care outside of the system, they'd be able to.

• • •

A few last thoughts on putting patients first …

Computerized health records, databases, and the internet are great tools for doctors, of that there is no debate. But these things can just as easily turn into a barrier between doctor and patient when it comes to providing quality health care. Physicians who've embraced technology and switched over from paper files to electronic medical records, for instance, too often spend their time with patients looking at the computer screen. Not only is this a real turnoff for the patient, it's also changed the way doctors diagnose problems. You've probably heard the expression, "The eyes are the gateway to the soul." Well, if you're a doctor, a patient's eyes can also give you a clue as to what's going on with them. However, if you're too busy typing, or looking something up on the internet, or trying to figure out what's the least expensive thing you can try first in order to help the government continue to ration health care, there's a real possibility you're going to mess up. Putting patients first, of course, would put an end to this. But unless our elected officials are willing to get serious about truly reforming our health care system, then we're going to continue on like this, underdiagnosing, overdiagnosing, and misdiagnosing — dealing only with symptoms and providing "episodic care" instead of trying to find the root cause of what's really going on with the patient — putting everyone's health at risk and coming ever closer to driving the fiscal bus over the cliff.

What's Stopping Us from Doing So?

Remember those kids who used to sit at the back of the classroom? The troublemakers? The slow learners? The social misfits? Well, guess what? They're the ones in charge now. Slowly but surely, bit by bit, the best and the brightest, who used to run for office, form governments, and be part of cabinets — federally and provincially — have been replaced by the very ones who sat at the back of the classroom. Canada is presently being governed by a prime minister who brings to the table perhaps the *thinnest* resumé we've ever seen from someone occupying that office. While our "Teflon PM" is admittedly photogenic and personable, one can't help getting the impression that if you scratched the surface you'd find there wasn't much there.

Sadly, things aren't much better at the provincial level. When you think back to the 1970s and 1980s, when people like Allan Blakeney, Bill Davis, Peter Lougheed, and Frank McKenna were heading up the provinces of Saskatchewan, Ontario, Alberta, and New Brunswick respectively, and then compare them to most of today's premiers, you can't help noticing there's been a hell of a drop-off in the talent department. Too many of them aren't true leaders — they're pretenders. They want us to believe they are nation builders, but what they really are is part of a demolition crew. Most don't understand the basic truth that for every action there is a *re*action. That if you're going to engage in social engineering, trying to solve poverty on the backs of businesses and physicians, then you're ultimately going to fail and the whole shithouse is going to come tumbling down. This is why it's so important that we stand up and speak out and not sit idly by while they puff and preen and blow out their cheeks, all in hopes of distracting us from what a bunch of failures they are.

"Prime Minister Selfie," as I like to refer to Justin Trudeau, and the aforementioned "do-gooder" premiers continue to put forward dopey ideas and interventionist policies that are designed to do one thing and one thing only: hide the truth from Canadians for as long as possible. The reality is, when it comes to health care, we can no longer afford to waste any more time. People need to know the truth. And what is that truth? It's quite simple. No one — I repeat, *no one* — is putting patients first in 2019, despite what name they might give to a particular piece of legislation. Unless we, as Canadians and as users of our health care system, start demanding better from those in charge — demanding specifically that they stop trying to impose all this crazy ideology on us and start putting patients first — then I'm afraid we're doomed to see medicare swirl down the drain of mediocrity for some time to come.

Surely, we can do better than this.

3. Revise the Canada Health Act So that "Quality" Becomes the Sixth Principle

If we don't soon start taking things seriously and make quality "Job One," instead of "Job None," the aforementioned iceberg that's lurking just below the surface will rip our health care system to shreds, putting our parents, ourselves, our children, and our children's children at risk. Think I'm kidding? Here's what the future holds if we continue to pretend we have the best health care system in the world and don't give a rat's ass about quality.

According to the *Daily Mail*, family doctors in England are receiving bonuses for putting patients on "death lists" in order to cut down on the number of bed-blockers in hospitals — seniors and those who can't look after themselves, who'd otherwise be in nursing homes if only there wasn't such a shortage of long-term-care beds. Doctors can even receive bonuses for drawing up end-of-life advanced care plans for those patients they figure will die within a year. According to a National Health Service internal memo, a key objective of the project is to "shift the place of death" away from hospitals, thereby "reducing health-care costs."

Or how about this?

Local county councils — again in England (and again as reported by the *Daily Mail*) — are putting the elderly and infirm up for auction on eBay-style websites, where nursing homes can bid against each other and offer them a bed. Naturally, the cheapest bid is the one that wins. Patients and their families have no say in the matter and are forced to relocate their loved ones to whichever nursing home won the bidding, sight unseen. This strategy has apparently reduced health care costs by a fifth.

But England has nothing on Greece, where the country's shaky finances have led to the dismantling of its health care system. As a result, according to the *New York Times*, patients who're hospitalized in Greece must hire their own nurses just to receive basic care. Except those black-market nurses aren't really nurses at all. They're mostly illegal immigrants, who work for temp agencies and who pose as family members in order to sneak into the patient's room and provide questionable care at a vastly reduced rate.

I could go on but I won't, as I think you're beginning to get the picture.

How Might We?

Here's the definition of health care quality you'll find if you go to the Health Quality Ontario website: "Health care quality is achieving better health outcomes and experiences for every person living in Ontario. Because better has no limit." Sounds good, doesn't it? I mean, who couldn't agree with a definition like that? And while I cringe to think how many taxpayer dollars were given to some advertising agency to come up with the "because better has no limit" slogan, I'm willing to set that aside for a moment and give the Ontario government full marks for determining there was a need for something like Health Quality Ontario in the first place. Exploring HQO's website a little further, one can't help being impressed by its mandate. "As the province's advisor on health care quality," we are told, "Health Quality Ontario has been entrusted to: monitor and report on how the health system is performing, provide guidance on important quality issues, assess evidence to determine what constitutes optimal care, engage with patients and give them a voice in shaping a quality health system, [and] promote continuous quality improvement aimed at substantial and sustainable positive change in health care."

Digging a little deeper, we come upon a document entitled *Quality Matters: Realizing Excellent Care for All*. This, we are led to believe, is a blueprint for a health care system that is safe, effective, patient-centred, timely, efficient, and equitable. For instance: "When a patient receives the right treatment, at the right time, and in the right setting, that is health care quality. When health care providers in different settings are able to work together in the best interest of the patient, that is health care quality. When system funders and institutions have the information they need to make good policies, that is health care quality. But how well do these aspirations stack up against reality?"

Ah, yes. The $64,000 question.

The document goes on to say that while various surveys have shown roughly three-quarters of Ontarians give the province's health care system high marks and that Ontario has no shortage of committed champions making a difference, the fact remains not all is well. Study after study published on the state of Ontario's health care system, we learn, reveals a system that is neither equitable nor sustainable. We also discover there's a pattern of gaps in health care, gaps that ultimately have significant negative consequences for patients. These include difficulty accessing primary care, long waits for specialty care, critical safety events in health care institutions, and poor access to medically necessary prescription medicine.

"Given this evidence," the document explains, "the unmistakable conclusion is that the Ontario health system works well for some people, with some conditions, treated in some institutions, at some points in time. That's situational quality, not systemic quality." A few paragraphs later, the authors of *Quality Matters: Realizing Excellent Care for All* make this rather startling admission: "In Ontario, there is neither a common understanding of what defines high quality care nor a road map to get from the status quo to the desired future."

How might we change all this, so that our health care system — Canada's, not just Ontario's — is committed to delivering high quality care at a price we can all afford? Health Quality Ontario suggests we do it by reinventing our health care system so it: (1) focuses on improving access for all sectors in a way that reflects the patient journey; (2) is concerned with preventing illness just as much as with treating it; (3) is accessible to all, regardless of who you are or where you live; (4) is responsive to the needs of the patients; (5) achieves a balance among competing priorities, recognizing the needs to address both quick wins and longer-term goals that are hard to achieve; (6) does not depend upon the infusion of new funding but instead redistributes resources to where they'll have the greatest impact; and (7) allows for fundamental change by removing barriers to innovation.

All sensible suggestions. But the question remains: "How do we get there from here?"

Why Would We Want To?

Why is quality so important? And why do I think we should revise the Canada Health Act so that quality becomes the sixth principle? Let me share a few stories with you that I believe illustrate my point rather well.

In January of 2016, a teenager by the name of Laura Hillier died while waiting for a stem-cell transplant. She was only eighteen years old and had her whole life ahead of her. Unfortunately for Laura, she made the mistake of getting sick in Ontario, a province where — like most of the rest of Canada — we've had our heads buried in the sand for far too long when it comes to how we fund our health care system. This young girl died not because they couldn't find a donor — there actually was one — but because the system couldn't find a way to fund the procedure that would've saved her life. Then there's little Meghan Arnott, a young girl who was waiting for surgery in British Columbia to correct a complication brought on by Crohn's disease. Meghan was told her surgery would likely have to be postponed eight or nine months because of a severe shortage of nurses in British Columbia, caused by — you guessed it — chronic underfunding of our health care system by the government. As a result, Meghan was forced to wait in excruciating pain and discomfort, yet another invisible victim of medicare. Or how about Walid Khalfallah, who hails from Kelowna, British Columbia? Walid is now a paraplegic thanks to his encounter with our health care system. All because those running the show felt it was a reasonable risk for a young boy of thirteen to wait twenty-seven months — that's right, I said *twenty-seven months* — for surgery on his spine. By the time Walid had the surgery in 2012, at Shriners Hospital in Spokane, Washington, it was too late.

My own story is equally as instructive.

It began innocently enough, as mentioned earlier, on a relatively pleasant early spring day in April of 2015. I had just finished walking the dogs, and was getting ready to go to a meeting, when I suddenly felt something going on with my heart. At first, I wasn't particularly alarmed. After all, this had happened before, which is why I was on medication to keep my particular problem — atrial fibrillation — under control. Hell, I'd even undergone a procedure four or five years earlier called a catheter ablation. This involves a doctor inserting a couple of long, thin tubes into a hole made in your groin and then guiding them up through your blood vessels, all the way to your heart. Electrodes on the tip of the tubes are then used to take care of any "hot spots," which are areas of your heart that fire so rapidly that its upper chambers quiver instead of beating normally. But it soon became apparent to me that this event was something different. After five or ten minutes of trying to ride out the storm, I woke my better half and told her she better call 911.

To make a long story short, the paramedics came to our house and took me to the local hospital, where I immediately lost consciousness and had to have my heart shocked back into rhythm by the emergency room doctors. When I came to, I saw the worried faces of my loved ones, who'd followed the ambulance in a cab. Despite their looks of concern, I figured it was better meeting them than meeting my maker. It was soon determined I'd had a V-tach attack and that I'd have to be transferred to a hospital in Toronto to receive the appropriate treatment.

I spent three days in hospital, where the specialists poked and prodded me, but couldn't figure out why this had happened. Had I missed my medication that morning? Did the cold pill I took that day before going to my meeting somehow set things off? Was there something wrong with my heart genetically? One specialist in particular was keen to put in some kind of pacemaker but a colleague talked him out of it and suggested more tests be done first. The specialist told me it might take several days or even weeks to get the tests. There was a wait-list. And this was Ontario. As a small-business owner — and the sole breadwinner for my family — I was faced with a difficult decision. Lie around in bed for God knows how long, waiting to find out what was wrong with me, or have the doctor discharge me and hope the tests could be arranged for me as an outpatient.

Not surprisingly, I chose the latter. Then waited in limbo for a year, until my number came up, and I was finally able to take those tests.

What's Stopping Us from Doing So?

How did it ever come to this? How did supposedly intelligent men and women, given the responsibility for running our health care system, allow things to deteriorate so badly? More importantly, how did we — the public — ever allow ourselves to be duped all these years? Stories like those of Laura, Meghan, and Walid, while admittedly anecdotal, make it clear Canada's health care system is no longer something we Canadians can — or should — be proud of. When you read about these kinds of encounters with our health care system, it's enough to make your blood boil. How can we even pretend to have the best health care system in the world? We're so far from being the best no one could possibly make that claim anymore with a straight face. Undoubtedly, there are serious inadequacies in how medicare is funded and how decisions are made when it comes to deciding which programs receive funding and which don't. It's sort of like winning the lottery. If you belong to a demographic that's older and more inclined to vote, then you might well be in luck. If you happen to be a child, though, or suffering from some less-than-"sexy" disease, then good luck, you're on your own.

No one's life should have to depend on a roll of the dice.

It took my own encounter with medicare back in 2015 to put things in perspective. When you're truly sick and facing a life-threatening situation, most of the time Canada's health care system has no equal. Imagine, for instance, that you're a race car driver at the Indianapolis 500 and you pull into the pits, where an incredible crew works on your car and gets you ready to get back out there. Everyone working in unison, everyone pulling together. That's our health care system at its best. Unfortunately, if it's not a "life or death" situation, if you're not about to expire, then our health care system is more like when a large Canadian city gets hit by a snowstorm — a really big one, say. Sure, highways and main streets get plowed within hours of the snow falling, but side streets may not be touched for several days. And that's the problem. Because our system is crumbling, and remains standing only as a result of the phenomenal dedication of our doctors and nurses and other health care professionals, people like me are forced to walk about like ticking time bombs, waiting for something bad to happen, so we can be rushed to the emergency department and receive the care we need when we need it from that wonderful pit crew.

I stated earlier that we'd be wise to adopt Ford's "Quality Is Job One" mantra. That might seem like a rather arbitrary borrowing, but what you may not know is just how many parallels there are between Canada's health care system and the automotive industry. For example, before Ford began his "Quality Is Job One" campaign in the summer of 1981, "Job One" meant something different in Detroit. The priority back then could be summed up in one simple sentence: "Don't worry about what the car is like, just get it out on time." The goal was clearly to get it off the assembly line, no matter what. Quality was seen as a low priority — just as it's been for the past fifty years here in Canada when we're talking about medicare. But as a result of some inspired thinking by Ford's president at the time, Philip Caldwell, who'd written a note to himself in 1978 that read, "quality — number one," the game was changed, and quality became the new priority for the automaker.

Bottom line: if we're ever going to have a health care system that actually works and delivers the kind of care Canadians need and deserve, then we're going to have to get a lot more serious about quality. It can't continue to be an afterthought. I've suggested it be added to the Canada Health Act as a sixth principle … but really, quality should be the *first* principle, as far as I'm concerned. Otherwise, we're just throwing good money after bad. And nobody wants that.

4. Combine All of Canada's Provincial and Territorial Health Ministries into One Federal "Super Ministry" with One Health Minister

It's quiz time. How many ministries of health do we currently have in Canada? Believe it or not, the answer is fourteen — ten provincial, three territorial, and one federal. Each province and territory has a health minister and a health ministry chock full of civil servants, most of whom never see a patient. That's a hell of a lot of dollars being spent on things other than frontline patient care. Imagine if we took all those bureaucracies and rolled them into one "super ministry," with one health minister and one bureaucracy — all located in Ottawa. The savings would be enormous.

Now, I understand this would involve making changes to Canada's Constitution — currently, the federal government writes the cheques and the provinces and territories deliver the care — but just think how much better off we'd be if the prime minister and premiers all agreed to do this. Take pharmaceuticals, for instance. How much sense does it make to have all these different provincial and territorial health ministries negotiating separate deals with Big Pharma? Is it any wonder the cost of prescription medicines is eating up so much of our health care budgets? Surely, the time has come for the piper to call the tune. The federal government can't just sit by and be a passive player anymore. In addition to providing the funding, it also needs to get its hands dirty and actually run our health care system — no matter how much the provinces and territories might kick and scream.

How Might We?

In the late 1980s, the Liberal government, under David Peterson, was looking to curry favour with rural Ontario and decided to develop a new program that would help farmers who'd suffered significant crop losses as a result of bad weather. I was asked to help with that program. My supervisor told me that first day that "everything was up in the air," that they "weren't really sure what they wanted," but that I'd probably be creating "some kind of form that farmers could use to apply to the new program." If you think this sounds like a recipe for disaster, you're right. I spent six months designing, revising, redesigning, and then revising once again a single form — all at $20 an hour (in 1980s dollars, remember). As it turns out, the crop insurance program was cancelled and all my hard work was for naught. On my way out the door, I could only watch in disbelief as the many thousands of copies of the form I'd spent the last six months slaving over were, rather unceremoniously, shredded.

I tell this story not as an indictment of government waste and foolishness but instead as a way of helping you understand the kind of culture we're dealing with here. Government is all about the here and now. Yesterday is gone and tomorrow is a long way away — that's pretty much the attitude. This is why I can't help laughing any time I hear some neophyte leader of a political party say that if they're elected, they'll clean up this mess and run government like a business. Good luck with that. No, a better idea would be to try to break down all those silos and get the different branches of government to actually *talk* to each other. Remember that line from *Cool Hand Luke*? "What we've got here is failure to communicate." Having spent the better part of the past quarter-century dealing with government and politicians, I can say with some degree of authority a lack of communication is the number one problem with how decisions are made and policy is developed. You've heard, of course, the old expression: "The right hand doesn't know what the left is doing." Well, that pretty much sums up how governments of all political stripes operate. This is why, if we're ever going to do something about fixing Canada's health care system, we need to wake up — and wake up soon — and admit we have a huge communications problem on our hands.

While my solution might be considered radical by some — recommending we combine all of Canada's provincial and territorial health ministries into one federal super ministry with one health minister — the truth is it's the only thing that makes sense. As illustrated by my crop insurance story, not knowing where you're going pretty much guarantees you won't know if and when you get there. Having the federal government write the cheques without having any involvement in how the provinces run our health care system is like filling up your car's gas tank and giving your kid the keys without first finding out whether or not he or she knows anything about how a car works or even if they know how to drive in the first place.

How nuts is that?

Why Would We Want To?

Imagine, if you will, how well medicare might function if we actually had a little leadership for a change. It speaks volumes that it took a provincial premier — Saskatchewan's Tommy Douglas — to grab the proverbial bull by the horns and show the rest of the country how we might provide health care for our citizens here in Canada. Had this been America, you can rest assured it wouldn't have been a governor leading the charge. It would've been the president. Remember John F. Kennedy? His historic speech in 1961 in which he promised the United States would land a man on the moon and bring him home safely before the end of the decade is precisely the sort of thing I'm talking about. Kennedy was a giant. So was Pierre Trudeau, as were Margaret Thatcher and Ronald Reagan. Sadly, all the giants are gone.

These days, we're being led by a bunch of followers.

This is, if we're to be honest about it, the problem. You can't lead from the middle. Building a consensus is fine if you're looking to order a pizza. But if you wish to reinvent Canada's health care system, consensus simply isn't going to cut it. Someone has to take charge. Someone has to speak truth to power. This is why I believe it's crucial that whoever sits in the prime minister's office following the next federal election must invite our country's provincial and territorial leaders to come to the table so we can finally have that adult conversation everyone keeps talking about. You know the one I mean. The one where we finally admit our health care system is no longer sustainable, that the status quo is no longer an option, and that it's time for some real, concrete solutions instead of playing make-believe.

Bottom line: fourteen health ministries is thirteen health ministries too many. Having seen first-hand how government functions, how civil servants run around trying to figure out how to please their political masters by telling them what they think they want to hear, and watching time and time again how politics wrecks good public policy, I have to tell you I don't hold out a lot of hope this can be done. I mean, it's not for nothing our health care system is the train wreck it is. Let me give you an example. In Ontario, the highly unpopular Wynne government, facing long odds and desperate to find some way of getting re-elected in order to continue its "legacy," hit upon a rather novel idea. "OHIP+," they called it. Under this plan, children and young adults, twenty-four years of age and younger, would have all their prescriptions covered by the Ontario government. Sounds like a wonderful idea, doesn't it? Until you look a little closer and discover the vast majority of those prescriptions were already being covered by the kids' parents' drug plans. Developing policy based on increasing your electoral success is wrong. Precious taxpayer dollars should never be wasted this way.

But in Canada's largest province, in 2018, they were. Fortunately, Doug Ford, who replaced Wynne as premier following the June election, righted this wrong and dramatically modified OHIP+.

If we had only one health ministry, however, it would be harder for self-serving politicians like Kathleen Wynne to hijack it. For instance, instead of thirteen different provinces and territories negotiating thirteen different deals with the pharmaceutical companies, Ottawa's super ministry could sit down and hammer out *one* deal for the entire country. Imagine how many millions — if not *billions* — of dollars that would save. And while we're at it, imagine the savings governments Canada-wide would enjoy if our bloated health care bureaucracy was cut in half — maybe even by three-quarters. I once tried to figure out how much Ontario's ministry of health and long-term care had grown back in the early 2000s. After discovering there was no easy way to figure this out, I had someone take two Ontario government phone books — one from 2001 and one from 2005 — and compare the number of phone extensions. Working on the assumption there'd likely be one employee for each extension, we estimated the bureaucracy of this particular ministry had *doubled* in five years.

What's Stopping Us from Doing So?

Of course, in order to roll all of our provincial and territorial health ministries into one super ministry, we'd need to open up Canada's Constitution and make a few changes. Right now, the way our Constitution is configured, the federal government is responsible for funding our health care system only. The provinces and territories get to decide how to design and run their individual systems — sort of like mini-fiefdoms — while following some rather basic and general guidelines set down by the feds. Under the system I'm proposing, everything would be different. The federal government would no longer be just "the banker," as if we were all playing some sort of perverse game of Monopoly.

The problem with opening up the Constitution, as I'm sure you're only too well aware, is that the provinces and territories wouldn't be content to deal with just health care. Quebec, which didn't sign on to Canada's Charter of Rights and Freedoms back in 1982, would surely use this opportunity to place some kind of demands upon the rest of the country. And who knows what the four western provinces might want? More control over their natural resources? Who can say? Still, in spite of these admittedly significant hurdles to overcome, I honestly believe that when men and women of good will get together, anything is possible — especially when it comes to fixing our broken health care system. After all, just about every province and territory is currently spending close to half of its annual budget on medicare.

Now, I'm not naive enough to think everyone involved in this process would have no problem checking their ego at the door. Elected officials, typically, covet one thing and one thing only — power. Some are lucky and seize power early. Others spend years chasing that Holy Grail. Either way, no politician worth their salt is likely to give up power without a fight — or, at the very least, without some sort of trade-off. If the provincial and territorial leaders are going to give up the right to run Canada's health care system, they're going to want something of significance back from the feds. And this is the problem: Ottawa, unless I'm mistaken, would be reluctant to give up anything of worth to provinces and territories.

This is a shame, because combining the thirteen provincial and territorial health ministries into one super ministry is an idea whose time has come. It would save us money, it would lead to efficiencies, and, perhaps most important of all, it would allow for the kinds of creativity and innovation Canada's health care system so badly needs. Sure, the provinces and territories are going to feel slighted, like they've done something wrong. Although really, despite the fact that they've pretty much been able to do whatever they want when it comes to health care for the past fifty years, the real blame lies with how medicare was constructed in the first place. If you're going to give your kid (the provinces and territories) a credit card with no limit and send them out there so they can spend like drunken sailors, then guess what? Eventually, dad (the federal government) is going to be left with little choice but to take the card away. That time, for better or worse, has finally arrived.

Deal with it.

5. Stop Focusing On Illness and Figure Out How to Keep Us Healthy Instead

Here's a dirty little secret that's not much of a secret. Our health care system has little to do with health. It's mostly about funding the treatment of those who're sick. Politicians like to pay lip service to the idea of keeping people healthy and helping them avoid hospitals, but it's really not much of a priority for them. This is unfortunate, because unless we start putting a little more time, money, and effort into wellness and prevention, we're not likely to survive the coming fiscal meltdown that will occur as a result of the obesity, diabetes, and dementia tsunamis waiting just around the corner.

So, what's my solution? Instead of burdening our health care providers with this, what I'd rather see is an expansion of the original ParticipACTION program from the 1970s, which was revived in 2007 after being a victim of budget cuts in 2001. Encouraging Canadians — especially our kids — to become more active, as well as teaching them about nutrition and the dangers of smoking, would go a long way toward lowering future health care costs. For the fact is, no matter how many millions we pour into medicare, no matter how many procedures we target, or goals we set, or wait-list websites we set up, unless we're willing to get serious about wellness and prevention, and actually try to do something about keeping people from getting sick in the first place, it'll all be for naught. We need to make this a priority.

How Might We?

Amazingly, you can still find it on YouTube — the original fifteen-second public service announcement that was meant to get Canadians off their collective butts. The ad shows two people jogging. One is wearing a red track suit, the other a blue track suit. We see the runners only from the waist down as the commercial begins. "These men are about evenly matched," the voice-over states. "That's because the average thirty-year-old Canadian is in about the same physical shape as the average sixty-year-old Swede." By this time, the camera has panned up to show the thirty-year-old Canadian runner huffing and puffing, while the sixty-year-old Swede is smiling and barely working up a sweat. "Run, walk, cycle," the voice-over continues. "Let's get Canada moving again." The ad, which ran during broadcasts of Canadian Football League games during the 1973 season, proved to be quite a sensation — even sparking a debate in the House of Commons in Ottawa.

Sadly, forty-six years later, not much has changed. A survey by the Heart and Stroke Foundation of Canada revealed that 60 percent of Canadians are overweight. Even worse, 25 percent of our kids are also too heavy. Although those numbers aren't as bad as the United States, where 69 percent of adults and 30 percent of children are overweight, when you factor in our body mass index, Canadians are among the fattest people on earth. As if that isn't bad enough, while 55 percent of adults say they engage in physical activity for at least thirty minutes a day, just one in four of our kids get the recommended one hour a day of exercise. Then there's our diet. The American Heart Association recently reported that less than 1 percent of Americans have a healthy diet. In Canada, that number is not much better. All this in spite of millions of dollars of advertising by governments at all levels in both countries. It's no wonder our health care systems are collapsing under the weight of all this. Our thumbs and fingers might be in excellent shape, thanks to all those video games we're playing — to mention nothing of our disturbing obsession with our smart phones and other electronic devices — but that's about it.

The Swedes, however, are still way ahead of us. While it's true Sweden's obesity rate is rising — don't get too excited; at 11 percent it's still only half of Canada's — where they have us beat six ways to Sunday is with their physical activity. The average Swede in the eighteen-to-thirty-nine-year-old category gets thirty-four minutes of daily activity, compared to the nineteen minutes on average the same cohort in Canada gets. Forget about Fit for Life. In Canada, too many of us are Fat for Life. Unless we wake up and make a serious commitment to staying active and eating right, then I'm afraid we'll discover just how unsustainable Canada's health care system truly is. Like a lifeboat with too many on board, our system will start to take on water and slowly begin to sink. We simply must take health and wellness more seriously. We need to teach our kids how to eat the right kinds of foods and the importance of staying active. And here, I'm not talking about blowing a bunch of money on lavish ad campaigns. While the shock value of something like the sixty-year-old Swede PSA might grab someone's attention for twenty or thirty seconds, what we really need is for every adult, every parent, every teacher, Scouter, and coach to connect with our kids, one on one, and explain why what most kids are doing to themselves is dangerous and that it'll hurt all of us down the road.

Health is wealth. That's a lesson well worth teaching to our children.

Why Would We Want To?

There's a black-and-white photograph my wife is especially fond of. It's a picture of my father holding me in his arms, while my mom stands by his side looking on lovingly. A crown of crazy curls adorns my head. A pair of chubby legs stick out of my shorts. Something must have distracted me just as the photo was being snapped, as my eyes are looking left, searching for God knows what. This particular snapshot — capturing a moment frozen in time — was taken in June of 1959, according to the date stamped on the back of the photo. That would make me six months old. Up in Ottawa, Dief was still the Chief. Down south, Ike and Dick were still clicking, although a handsome young Irish Catholic named Kennedy and his glamorous wife would soon be making headlines. Here in Toronto, Johnny Bower — the China Wall — was preparing for his second season as the Leafs' netminder.

Sixty years later, I can't help wondering where the time went.

Now, when I wake up in the morning, the first thing I have to figure out is whether or not I've died in the night. Once I'm convinced I've survived another night and live to face another day, I need to see if all my body parts are still functioning. I wiggle my toes, bend my knees, and then lift my arms heavenward. If everything seems to be in working order, I sit up and swing my legs over the side of the bed, trying hard to blink away the blurry vision, and see if I can feel the floor beneath my feet — or even feel my feet, which I often can't do. After sitting on the side of the bed for a minute or so, I try to stand without falling over. Sometimes I get "the spins" and have to grab onto something — the duvet, the blinds, air — to keep from toppling over. Finding my slippers, I do what my wife calls my "old man shuffle" to the bathroom, where I hobble over to the toilet and sit down again.

Like most baby boomers, my days are filled with pills and potions, liniments and ointments — all meant to manage pain, which to varying degrees they mostly do. My knees are shot, my ankles feel like someone's constantly jabbing them with a Ginsu knife, and my back is always aching. When I try to stand up straight, I'm told I look like those pictures of J.D. Salinger just before he died — an old man, nearly ninety then, bent at the waist, looking at the ground like he was hoping to find some change. But that's not the worst of it. The hair on my chest has all turned white, while my shins are so shiny you'd swear I was using Nair on them. I have more hair in my ears and nostrils than I have on my head — that's not entirely accurate, I know, but I do seem to spend more time shaving my ears and nose than any other body part. All that's bad enough, but I'm also thirty to forty pounds overweight and, judging by the size of my gut, I appear to have swallowed a basketball while I was sleeping.

It wasn't always this way, of course. Until I turned forty, I was mostly getting away with not exercising and eating like someone bent on committing suicide with food. But then things started going wrong. First of all, during a routine checkup, it was discovered my blood pressure was 160/120. Then I was felled with kidney stones and shortly thereafter a hernia. My doctor put me on medication for the high blood pressure and I underwent two medical procedures for the kidney stones, as well as surgery for the hernia. During a follow-up investigation, they found I had a huge cyst on my good kidney — the one without the stones. A nutritionist at the hospital asked me a few weeks after the kidney stones were broken down and flushed out of my system about my diet. "How much cheese do you eat?" she wanted to know. I gave her my best guess. "Is that a year, a month, a week?" she asked. "A day," I responded, sheepishly. "I can't understand how you're still alive," she said, shaking her head.

Me neither.

What's Stopping Us from Doing So?

In January of 2018, a study conducted by Dr. Daniel Dutton of the School of Public Policy at the University of Calgary was made public. The study's findings suggested the best way to ensure we have a healthier population is by spending more not on health care but on social services instead. "Spending more on health care sounds like it should improve health, but our study suggests that is not the case and social spending could be used to improve the health of everyone," Dr. Dutton said. "Relative to health care, we spend little on social services per person, so redistributing money to social services from health care is actually a small change in health care spending." The study examined data from nine of Canada's ten provinces over a thirty-one-year period, from 1981 to 2011, in hopes of determining whether or not there was a link between social and health care spending and poor health. Data revealed that average per capita spending on social services was $930, while $2,900 — almost three times the amount — was spent on providing health care services. Further, the study showed that health spending per capita had increased tenfold over the three decades the study covered when compared with spending on social services.

Focusing on three broad areas — potentially avoidable mortality, infant mortality, and life expectancy — Dr. Dutton's study revealed some rather surprising and unexpected findings. "Social spending as a share of health spending is associated with improvements in potentially avoidable mortality and life expectancy," Dr. Dutton said. "If governments spent one cent more on social services per dollar spent on health by rearranging money between the two portfolios, life expectancy could have experienced an additional 5 percent increase and potentially avoidable mortality could have experienced an additional 3 percent decrease in one year."

These findings are important because they represent some powerful new data those of us who hope to reinvent Canada's health care system can use in order to help us create something new and better. Clearly, "the same old same old" isn't working anymore. We need to dramatically change our way of thinking and stop flushing good money after bad down the drain. By adjusting how we allocate money to health care services and social services, we just might be able to improve the health of Canadians while not bank-rupting the country. "If social spending addresses the social determinants of health," Dr. Dutton went on to explain, "then it is a form of preventative health spending and changes the risk distribution for the entire population rather than treating those with disease. Redirecting resources from health to social services, that is, rearranging payment without additional spending, is an efficient way to improve health outcomes."

But before going down this road and making changes to how we allocate both health care and social services dollars, we need to keep a few things in mind. Firstly, medicare, as it was originally conceived by Tommy Douglas and Justice Emmett Hall, was never meant to deal with population health but was instead designed as a sort of "security blanket" to prevent Canadians from having to declare bankruptcy as a result of falling ill. Secondly, while in broad terms it may well make sense to redirect funding to help those at the lower end of the socio-economic scale, there's no practical way to predict what diseases or illnesses the poor are likely to find themselves dealing with. What'll likely happen in all probability is that politicians will continue to set up pricey programs targeting certain groups of voters in hopes of winning their votes come election time, because they know the underprivileged don't typically vote. Lastly, government being government, you just know that if such a program were to be set up and more dollars were allocated to social services, much of the expanded funding would go to cover the salaries and benefits of the army of civil servants who'd be hired to run such a program.

So, while Dr. Dutton's study is both useful and timely, it too will likely sit on a shelf somewhere, ignored by those who have the power to make a difference.

6. Open the Door to "Medical Tourism"

Funny thing. We seem to have no problem offering up our expertise and technologies to the rest of the world in other fields. So why do we suddenly get all queasy when we talk about doing the same thing when it comes to health care? Obviously, the situation we find ourselves in calls for a little creativity. Especially when you consider the fact that we're currently spending over $200 billion annually on health care here in Canada. This breaks down to nearly $6,000 for every man, woman, and child. Why not turn medicare into a revenue generator? Why not make it something more than just a cost centre? It'd help create good-paying jobs in the health care sector and would boost local economies, especially those with hotel rooms and luxury suites sitting half empty most of the year. And a portion of the fees could go toward filling government coffers. If our leaders truly care about ensuring that medicare is sustainable in the years to come, then embracing "medical tourism" could well be an excellent way to go about it.

Sound crazy?

Well, just imagine an advertising campaign — sometime down the road — that boldly proclaims, "Come to Toronto (or Montreal, or Vancouver, or Calgary, or Halifax) to get your hip (or knee) replacement (or heart bypass, or double lung transplant), where the scalpels are sharp, the operating rooms are clean, and the weather is fine!" This can be the future of medicare, if only we have the courage to be bold and imaginative visionaries.

A few provisos, though: One, these services should be offered only in private health care facilities and not government-run, publicly funded hospitals. This would ensure no Canadian patient would ever be "bumped" so that a foreign patient with money, who's willing to pay, could jump the public queue. Two, before opening the door to medical tourism, every Canadian must be granted the right to purchase private health insurance and access private care throughout all of Canada — not just Quebec — without any restrictions. Three, if the government can't provide the appropriate care for a patient in a timely fashion, then it should be morally and legally obligated to send that patient to one of these private clinics, using public dollars to cover the costs.

How Might We?

In 2017, the Fraser Institute released a report estimating that some sixty-three thousand Canadians had travelled outside the country to seek medical care the previous year. This represented a 40 percent increase over the previous year and was thought to be as a result of long wait times for medical procedures in Canada. Because there were no reliable data on which to base their report, the Fraser Institute was forced to rely on its own surveys. The think tank polled a number of Canadian physicians, representing twelve specialities, including cardiovascular surgery, neurosurgery, oncology, orthopaedic surgery, and urology. Respondents were asked to provide their best estimate as to the number of their patients who received non-emergency treatment outside the country in the previous twelve months. Based on responses from those polled, the Fraser Institute came up with the number of 63,459. Of those, nearly 9,500 had travelled abroad for general surgery, another 6,400 went for urological treatments, and a further 5,000 went somewhere other than Canada in hopes of finding quicker access to colonoscopies and angiograms. Digging even deeper, we discover that 26,513 of these patients came from Ontario, 15,372 from British Columbia, and 9,067 from Alberta.

Yanick Labrie, a senior fellow at the Fraser Institute and one of the authors of the report, said, "If that many Canadians are willing to pay out of pocket to get faster access to the treatment they need, that means they are dissatisfied with the quality of care." But Jeremy Snyder, a professor at Simon Fraser University's faculty of health sciences disagreed with the report's conclusions that Canada has a growing problem with medical tourism as a result of ever-increasing wait times at home. While we know a lot of Canadians are going aboard for care, Dr. Snyder explained, in his view the numbers the Fraser Institute came up with aren't really accurate, noting that there's no real evidence to support the theory that Canadians are being forced to go elsewhere simply because of long wait times at home.

But Hector Macmillan, a former mayor of Trent Hills, Ontario, took umbrage with Professor Snyder's remarks, calling the Fraser Institute's report "damning." Macmillan, diagnosed with pancreatic cancer in January of 2016, and who'd hoped to undergo a NanoKnife procedure in the United States, had begged Ontario's ministry of health and long-term care to pay for the operation. When the Ontario Health Insurance Program denied Macmillan's request, he went to Germany instead, after raising the necessary funds on his own. "Our health care system is certainly broken," Macmillan told reporters upon his return to Canada. "I think it's time for a total overhaul." After publicly embarrassing Ontario's health minister, Dr. Eric Hoskins, in a public forum, asking the minister why he was willing to let him die, Hector Macmillan managed to persuade the Ontario government to conduct a clinical trial to see if the NanoKnife procedure should be covered for Canadians seeking cancer treatment outside the country. Unfortunately for Macmillan, he died in 2017 without knowing whether his extraordinary efforts to convince the government to show a little more compassion toward those facing a death sentence from cancer were worth it or not.

Evidently, there is a market — if not a genuine need — for Canadians seeking treatment elsewhere. "Public health care in Canada is seen as a bit of a religion," Raffi Elliott, a self-styled health care entrepreneur based in Armenia, told thousands of attendees at a medical tourism conference in Ottawa in 2016. "But it has its shortfalls and a lot of people end up falling through the cracks." Guillaume Debaene, general manager of Vancouver-based MediTravel International, agreed, saying, "[Medical travel] is becoming more and more popular for Canadians. However, millions of them still don't know what it is exactly and that it is available as a possible solution to them."

But what if, instead of sending people out of the country to seek treatment elsewhere, they could stay right here? Even more importantly, what if Canada became a destination for medical tourists? Let's take a look at how we might do both.

Why Would We Want To?

When Kevin Falcon, at the time British Columbia's health minister, first raised the idea of promoting the province as a destination for medical tourism, he was somewhat surprised by the amount of pushback from those who were opposed to the idea. Rising in the B.C. legislature in May of 2010, he informed members he'd been speaking with a number of physicians — particularly surgeons — who'd made it clear the province shouldn't just look at health care as a cost, but rather as a revenue generator that could potentially bring in millions of dollars to B.C.'s treasury, which could then be reinvested into the health care system. "Take all those Americans who seek treatment elsewhere every year," Falcon told the legislature. "You could charge these individuals enough that you could not only cover the costs of the operation or whatever the elective surgical procedure may be, but you could also have enough to plow back into the system to provide quicker and better access for British Columbians that may be on elective wait lists."

By relaxing the rules and opening the door to innovation, Falcon concluded, there's no reason British Columbia couldn't become the Mayo Clinic of the north.

Not surprisingly, the defenders of the status quo and other naysayers had plenty of reasons why this was a bad idea. Alice Edge, co-chair of the B.C. Health Coalition, in an op-ed said Falcon's idea was "a non-starter." "We need to build on the proven public innovations that make this system stronger," Edge wrote, "and not be distracted by marketing schemes dressed up as public policy." A couple of years later, in 2012, Leigh Turner, an associate professor at both the University of Minnesota's Center for Bioethics and its School of Public Health, wrote in *Healthcare Policy*, "Canadians should tell their elected representatives to 'Hold the Mayo' and not waste public resources on efforts to attract international patients to provincial healthcare systems that already face many challenges in providing Canadians with timely access to medically necessary care." As a result of this backlash, this excellent initiative was soon spiked, and Kevin Falcon found himself on the outside looking in. "At this time, the ministry is not considering a plan to market health care services to individuals outside our province," a ministry of health spokesperson told the media in 2017. "Our priority at this time is to improve access to care for British Columbians and to ensure that they are able to access the care they need as close to home as possible."

Fortunately, support for the idea of turning Canada into an international destination for medical tourists is growing. In a recent report released by the Global Healthcare Policy and Management Forum, it was pointed out that as a result of trade agreements that allow people from various countries to access health care services elsewhere, the globalization of health care has been expanding, not decreasing. "Medical tourism has been taken up by governments as an economic growth engine," the report said, "with potential for generating and diversifying employment opportunities in struggling regional economies, boosting demand for locally-produced medical equipment and attracting biotechnology research and development." The authors of the report went on to say that while data on the indirect economic impacts of medical tourism are scarce, the most significant economic benefits may well be for non-medical sectors. In other words, not only would Canada's health care system benefit by entering this brave new world and embracing medical tourism, our hospitality industry and others would reap huge rewards, as well. While countries in Asia, Latin America, and the Middle East aggressively promote medical tourism and build facilities specifically to attract and serve international patients, Canada dawdles and doodles, wasting opportunities and falling further behind.

The numbers pretty much say it all — and it's not a pretty story. In 2013, for example, Canadians travelling abroad to receive medical treatment spent $447 million. Now compare that with the $150 million spent on accessing Canadian health care services by foreign visitors in the same year and you can see we have a huge trade imbalance here. Of course, it doesn't have to be that way. Our country is uniquely positioned — as a result of our proximity to the United States, which, don't forget, boasts the world's largest economy — to become a world leader in the field. All it would take is the political will to make it happen and a bang-up marketing campaign to let the world know that, when it comes to medical tourism, Canada is open for business.

What's Stopping Us from Doing So?

Of course, Canada wouldn't be Canada if we didn't keep coming up with new and inventive ways to "miss an opportunity to miss an opportunity." Forget the beaver — our country's national symbol should be the mule. We're so stubborn and intransigent. Take Colleen Flood, for instance. Flood, a professor in the University of Ottawa's Centre for Health Law, Policy and Ethics, argues that allowing foreigners to pay for health care treatment in Canada might actually be a bad thing because it would make our access to care problems even worse for Canadians. "Even if there is some reinvestment back that measurably benefits public patients," Professor Flood wrote in an article for *Policy Options*, "this has to be traded off against the fact that beds for medical tourists are clearly beds that could be used — right now — by Canadians."

Not content to stop there, Professor Flood goes on to suggest that any aggressive expansion of medical tourism in Canada would eventually have a negative effect on our public health care system by pulling doctors into the private system as a result of the irresistible lure of filthy foreign lucre. She also claims any perceived inefficiencies in Canada's current health care system won't be addressed by an influx of international money. "With respect to wait times," the good professor concludes, "research tells us that we won't solve this problem with more private dollars." What research and why not? As usual, whenever the prophets of doom and gloom speak, my skin starts to crawl. It's like listening to the screech of fingernails on a chalkboard. As unpleasant an experience as I can think of.

No, I'd much rather listen to the voice of reason — someone like Gwyn Morgan, a nationally recognized Canadian business leader and top executive, who frequently writes on health care. Here's what he had to say about the state of Canada's health care system in 2017. "Almost every Canadian has a family member or friend suffering on ever-lengthening wait lists," Morgan wrote in a *Financial Post* op-ed. "That's the human toll."

But what about the economic and social cost? Across Canada, health care consumes more than 40 percent of provincial revenues, reducing funds available for education, social programs, and infrastructure. Morgan goes on to say that a Fraser Institute study, "The Private Cost of Public Queues for Medically Necessary Care, 2017," revealed that the 973,505 Canadians waiting for treatment lost $1.7 billion in 2016 in wages alone. And this number would be twice as high if lost time before seeing a specialist after being referred by a general practitioner was also factored in. Taken together, those wait times averaged twenty weeks in 2016.

Referencing the aforementioned Fraser Institute study that showed more than sixty thousand Canadians had gone outside our country seeking treatment, Morgan summed it up far better than I ever could. "Herein lies an enormous economic opportunity," he wrote.

> So-called "medical tourism" is a huge and growing business. Third world countries such as India and Thailand attract thousands of foreign customers, including Canadians. Removing prohibitions against private care would reverse the flow of money going to international private hospitals, better utilize our world-class health care professionals and foster job-creating investment in one of the world's fastest growing sectors. Canada's universal no-charge public health care system would remain sacrosanct, while Canadians who choose to access the private clinics would help reduce both wait-times and costs.

Now that's *real* Canadian common sense, don't you think?

7. Invest Heavily in Long-Term Care — Or Be Prepared to Face the Consequences

Want to fix the "bed-blocker" problem in our hospital emergency departments? Start building more specialized nursing homes so all those seniors who can't take care of themselves and are stuck taking up valuable space — occupying hospital beds meant for acute-care patients, as opposed to long-term care ones — will finally have some place to go.

It's really that simple.

How Might We?

To fully appreciate the crisis our country is undergoing in long-term care, you must first understand how this crisis is affecting the day-to-day operations of Canada's acute-care hospitals — especially when it comes to overcrowding in their emergency departments. When the old and infirm have a health care crisis — or even just "an episode" — they often find themselves languishing in their local hospital's emergency department, waiting to go to a long-term care facility. Unfortunately, because a spot may not be available at just that precise moment, these people — grandma or grandpa, mom or dad, whoever it might be — end up being "bed-blockers." "Bed-blocker" is a term I personally hate and would like to see retired. I think that referring to these unfortunate souls as alternate level of care (or ALC) patients would be far better. Either way, no matter how you refer to them, they create myriad problems for hospital administrators — in particular, longer wait times to see a doctor in emergency departments. This results in a variety of poor outcomes for the trapped patient, especially seniors, including anything from accelerated functional decline, to social isolation, to loss of independence.

Researchers at the University of Waterloo and the Hamilton Niagara Haldimand Brant Community Care Access Centre took a closer look at the problem and discovered the following: although patients whose discharge was delayed because of a lack of space in nursing homes accounted for only 9 percent of the total number of patients with delayed discharge, they accounted for an astonishing 40 percent of delayed-discharge bed days. Or, to put it another way, those waiting for admission to long-term care facilities represent a relatively small portion of bed-blockers but block those beds for a much longer time than an average patient does. These findings are important because they show — in real terms — the costs of not doing something about our long-term care problem.

Even more alarming, those conducting this research project found that patients with the longest discharge delays inevitably exhibited one of four characteristics: morbid obesity, a psychiatric diagnosis, abusive behaviours, or stroke. This is important to our understanding of the problem we're facing, because it means that one-quarter of delayed-discharge days are caused by patients who cannot be easily cared for in most of Ontario's existing long-term care facilities. Remember, lifting and carrying patients from one location to another — even if just to the bathroom — is one of the leading causes of injury for personal support workers. Needless to say, the heavier the patient, the greater the risk of injury. And while many nursing homes are able to care for patients exhibiting signs of dementia, few are equipped to deal with those suffering from serious psychiatric disorders or those who are abusive to themselves and others. Which leaves us with stroke victims. True, many of these patients can regain some functionality with the appropriate care and rehabilitation, but, again, not all nursing homes have the ability to provide such therapies.

Clearly, simply spending more money to create more spaces in existing long-term care facilities is not the answer. And yet, that's what our leaders — at least in Ontario — have chosen to do. In 2017, Premier Kathleen Wynne laid out her government's vision — a twenty-point plan called Aging with Confidence — to help deal with the problem. The plan called for five thousand new long-term care beds by 2021–22, with a pledge to build a further twenty-five thousand beds over the next decade. Taking politics out of the equation for a moment, however, we see how wrong-headed this vision was. Given the challenges the aforementioned group of patients are facing, simply expanding the current system's capacity will do little to reduce the number of discharge delays our hospitals are having to deal with. What we should be doing instead is figuring out ways of designing nursing homes in such a way that they'll better able to accommodate the specialized needs of those patients who're plugging up the system. But we're not just talking "bricks and mortar." No, no, no. Our governments also need to invest in specialized training and equipment so those charged with the responsibility of caring for the elderly and infirm will actually have the tools and expertise required to do the job properly.

Why Would We Want To?

The situation in Canada's long-term care facilities is desperate. Taking the Province of Ontario during the years 2015 and 2016 as our example, it was reported by the Ontario Long Term Care Association that 97 percent of residents require assistance with daily activities such as getting out of bed, eating, or using the bathroom. A further 97 percent have two or more chronic conditions such as arthritis or heart disease. Ninety percent have some form of cognitive disease, while 46 percent exhibit some level of aggressive behaviour related to their cognitive impairment or mental health condition. Sixty-one percent take ten or more medications; 58 percent use a wheelchair; 40 percent have a mood disorder such as anxiety, depression, bipolar disorder, or schizophrenia; and 38 percent require around-the-clock monitoring for an acute medical condition.

A huge number of personnel and a massive amount of resources are needed to care for all of these people. And a coordinated system is needed to make sure that needs are met and that staff and resources are used efficiently. But, let's be honest about it. The way we provide long-term care for our seniors and most vulnerable citizens is little more than a dog's breakfast of programs, designed — again, if we're being truthful — to warehouse those we don't have time to deal with properly or whom we would rather forget even exist in the first place.

Don't believe me?

The following statistics, also provided by the Ontario Long Term Care Association, give us a sense of the enormity of the problem. As of June 2017, in Ontario, 625 homes were licensed and approved to operate as long-term care facilities in the province. Fifty-eight percent of these homes are privately owned, 23 percent are non-profit or charitable, and 16 percent are run by municipalities. Roughly 40 percent of Ontario's long-term care homes are small, with ninety-six or fewer beds. Of these, slightly less than half (47 percent) are located in rural communities. A total of 77,541 long-stay beds are allocated to provide care, accommodation, and services to frail seniors who require permanent placement. Five-hundred-forty-three convalescent-care beds are allocated to provide short-term care as a bridge between hospitalization and the patient's home. Three-hundred-fifty-nine beds are allocated to provide respite for families who need a break from caring for their loved ones 24/7.

Getting depressed yet? If not, then chew on these last few numbers for a moment.

Approximately three hundred of Ontario's long-term care facilities are older and need to be redeveloped — actions that will affect more than thirty thousand of the province's total number of long-term care beds. The average wait time for a patient to be successfully placed into long-term care, as of June 2017, was 137 days. The wait-list for long-stay beds — again, as of June 2017 — was 32,046. Drilling down even further, the *Hamilton Spectator* discovered the following as part of an investigative series they ran in 2017: roughly one in four long-term care residents in Ontario reported their pain is not well controlled, one in six was physically restrained at least once during the previous three-month period, one in five were being prescribed drugs experts say shouldn't be given to the elderly, and one in four newly admitted long-term care residents in Ontario found themselves being prescribed a class of sedatives known as benzodiazepines. Even more alarming, one in seven was being prescribed antipsychotic drugs without a clear rationale for doing so.

These numbers would seem to indicate we're either killing our loved ones by delaying their care or drugging to death those fortunate enough to find a long-term care facility. Small wonder one Ontario official expressed his frustration over the situation by exclaiming, "In Ontario, it's easier to get into a cemetery than find a bed in a long-term care home."

Then there is the issue of hands-on care. In Ontario, four hours of hands-on care per day is generally considered to be the minimum standard. Unfortunately, because of staffing and funding constraints, many homes only provide residents with somewhere between two and a half and three hours per day of direct care. The Ontario government disagrees with those figures, claiming long-term residents in the province receive an average of three and a half hours of direct care per day. However, the union representing long-term care workers says those numbers are way off because they include things like paid vacation days and sick leave in their calculations — situations where residents are obviously not receiving care.

Want one final distressing set of statistics? Of the almost eighty thousand people living in long-term care facilities in Ontario, the majority are over eighty-five years old, and almost three-quarters have some form of dementia, or mobility issues, or both.

We simply can't ignore this any longer. We have to do something about it.

What's Stopping Us from Doing So?

In her first report to the Ontario legislature in 2017, the province's patient ombudsman, Christine Elliott (who would be named deputy premier and minister of health and long-term care by Doug Ford the following year, after the PC party swept Kathleen Wynn's Liberals from power), reported that roughly 60 percent of the more than 1,500 complaints her office received during its first year of operation were a result of less-than-stellar communication from officials representing the hospital, long-term care, and home-care sectors. By far, the vast majority of those complaints had to do with patient discharges from hospitals — in particular, for those identified as alternate level of care patients. "We've heard of situations where people do feel pressured to make decisions," Ms. Elliott revealed to a roomful of reporters at a Queen's Park media conference, "and really don't feel that they're being treated as an individual or a human being — that they're just a number and a bed blocker and they need to be moving out."

Dr. Samir Sinha, director of geriatrics for two Toronto hospital networks and leader of Ontario's seniors' strategy, has a different take on the situation. "I don't think there are any hospitals trying to do bad things," she told reporters at the same media conference. "The challenge for hospitals is they are in the business of providing acute care. But when 15 percent of their beds on a daily basis are actually occupied by people that they can't help transition to a more appropriate setting, it creates stress on the system, it creates stress on the providers and it creates stress on families who are caught in the middle."

So, who's right — Christine Elliott or Dr. Sinha?

Actually, they both are. The hospitals aren't the villains here. Neither are the patients, the ones taking up space and occupying beds meant for acute-care patients or, even worse, languishing in hospital corridors. The real villains are … you guessed it. I can't tell you how many times over the past thirty years I've been forced to watch one exchange after another between party leaders and the premier, or health care critics and the health minister, regarding the ongoing problem of overcrowding in hospital emergency departments. Time and time again, the opposition hammers on the government, bringing up one individual case after another, pleading that they have to do something about the problem. And as often as not, after two or three days of bluff and bluster, someone from the front benches will inevitably rise in the legislature and announce they're going to make "an investment" in the health care of the people who reside in this province. Or to put it another way, they're going to throw money at the problem.

But will simply throwing money at this particular problem actually work? I can guarantee you it won't. Because, as I've said many times before, you can't fix the situation if you're trying to solve the wrong problem. Remember, politicians feel they have one job and one job only — and that's to do everything in their power to get themselves re-elected. Solving the problem of overcrowding in our emergency departments and finding a way to deal with the ever-worsening bed-blocker situation will take courage, commitment, and ingenuity. Three things history has shown us, over and over again, our elected officials are sorely lacking. No, it's going to take a revolt by us — the citizens of this country — to finally see some real change when it comes to taking care of the elderly and infirm. First and foremost, we, as a society, need to see a change in attitude. It's shameful the way we treat our seniors. The "me first" attitude that those in charge have been so quick to take advantage of has made it possible for us to think it's perfectly all right to "warehouse" our parents, our aunts and uncles, and even, in some cases, our siblings.

While out of sight may be out of mind for some, we'd all be wise to remember one thing. The time will come for all of us when we, too, will find ourselves facing the end. Alone, unloved, and forgotten is no way to do it.

8. Bring Back Co-payments and User Fees and Introduce Tax-Free Medical Savings Accounts

As previously mentioned, when the Patron Saint of Medicare, Tommy Douglas, brought in his version of public health care, he actually expected the citizens of Saskatchewan to pay out of their own pockets for a portion of the services they received. It just made sense. Regrettably, somewhere along the way politics once again got in the way of good public policy so that terms like "co-payments" and "user fees" came to be associated with the Devil — in this case, the United States of America.

Want to really fix our health care system for a generation, as Prime Minister Paul Martin claimed he was going to do back in 2004? Reintroduce co-payments and user fees. A measly $100 co-payment per annum for every man, woman, and child in Ontario, for instance, would generate over $1 billion worth of badly needed revenue. Want to fix the overcrowding problem in our hospital emergency departments? Charge everyone who goes there twenty-five dollars each time they walk through the doors. Visiting your family doctor? Ten bucks seems about right.

Harsh medicine, maybe. But necessary if we're going to have a health care system that future generations can rely upon.

And while we're at it, why not bring in tax-free medical savings accounts? The concept is pretty simple. Let the people decide what they'd like to spend their money on. After all, Canadians can already put away money for their retirement and their kids' education, so why not health care, too? Although not a cure-all, MSAs do have the potential to take a lot of pressure off medicare, acting as a safety valve, and likely reducing wait-lists. A single piece of legislation, allowing us to set aside up to $30,000 annually to cover any sort of health care services — medically necessary, or not — is all it would take.

Not exactly brain surgery, is it?

How Might We?

It never fails to amaze me just how many of my fellow Canadians mistakenly think our country's health care system is fully funded by our government. Maybe it's because of all the falsehoods, half-truths, and complete fabrications coming out of the mouths of our leaders. Or perhaps it's simply a case of "if you tell a lie often enough, people will begin to believe it." Truth be told, while 70 percent of Canada's health care services *are* financed by the federal government, a not-insignificant amount — 30 percent — is covered by other means. Fourteen-point-seven percent — or $29 billion — comes out of your pocket and mine, while most of the rest is covered by individual insurance plans, typically provided as part of a benefit package by an employer and covering such things as dental care, eye care, and prescription drugs.

Those in favour of bringing back user fees and co-payments — and I'm one of them — typically make the following argument. First and foremost, user fees and co-payments would go a long way toward helping fund our health care system. As you will see in a moment, our ability to continue to pay for even the most basic of health care services is being put at risk as a result of two factors — too many baby boomers accessing the system and not enough Gen-Xers and millennials to pay for it. The second argument in favour of user fees and co-payments is that many of us believe it would act as a deterrent and help eliminate some of those unnecessary visits to the emergency department by those who either don't have a family doctor of their own or who can't be bothered to wait a few days to get in to see their physician.

However, the introduction of user fees and co-payments by itself is not enough to cure what ails our health care system. We also need to offer Canadians choice — and that's where medical savings accounts come in. Medical savings accounts (or MSAs, for short) were first made available to self-employed individuals in the United States as a way of setting aside funds to pay for medical expenses — money that would be tax-deductible so long as it went toward paying for medical expenses not covered by any government plan. A similar program — bearing the name health savings accounts (or HSAs) — exists in Canada. Unfortunately, both MSAs and HSAs are available only to those running small businesses. What I'm proposing is that the Government of Canada introduce a medical savings account that would be available to all Canadians — not just those running a small business — similar to what we currently have, such as registered retirement savings plans (RRSPs), registered education savings plans (RESPs), and tax-free savings accounts (TFSAs).

It just makes sense, when you stop and think about it. If we can put away money for our retirement, or set aside funds for our children's education, or as a way of deferring tax to such a time as when we'll be taxed at a lower rate because of our age, why on earth can't we open up an account whose sole purpose is to help us pay for medical expenses while reducing the amount of tax we pay? After all, we seem to have no problem with people spending money on cigarettes, booze, cars, and big-screen television sets. So why does everyone get so bent out of shape when I suggest we grant those living in this country the right to set aside money in a medical savings account so they can spend it on health care in any way they see fit. For instance, let's say you need hip replacement surgery, or a kidney transplant, or cataract surgery, and you're not willing to wait, in pain, the many months or years it might take you to be treated here in Canada as a tax-paying citizen of this country. Why shouldn't you have the right to make a withdrawal from your MSA in order to pay for the health care services you can't get here in this country because our government refuses to either properly fund our health care system or to free it?

Good question.

Why Would We Want To?

Quick now. What do Australia, France, Germany, Italy, the Netherlands, New Zealand, Sweden, and Switzerland all have in common? Give up? Like Canada, they provide universal health care for their citizens. Unlike Canada, none of these countries prohibit the charging of user fees or co-payments. Instead, each and every one of them expects patients to share in the costs of providing health care and imposes either deductibles, or co-payments, or both on everyone — with the notable exceptions of the poor and the most vulnerable. Think about this for a moment. Like Canada, all eight of the aforementioned countries either fund health services via the tax system (e.g., Norway) or through government-provided insurance coverage (e.g., Germany). But, unlike Canada, none of these countries tie the funding of health care to some kind of sick, perverse ideal of patriotism. The reason, I believe, is pretty simple. The governments of Australia, France, Germany, Italy, the Netherlands, New Zealand, Sweden, and Switzerland have come to recognize that we're living in the twenty-first century. Health care systems that were developed and introduced in the 1960s — like Canada's health care system was — have been slow to adapt to demographic changes and inflationary realities.

Bottom line: either we accept this new reality and change, or we're doomed.

Think I'm kidding? Take a gander at these numbers for a moment. Eighteen- to twenty-four-year-olds in Canada face an unemployment rate of close to 20 percent. More than a quarter of those who are lucky enough to be employed are working part-time or in temporary jobs and their average household debt is $74,000. By not allowing user fees and co-payments, our country is asking this generation of Canadians to fund the health care costs of people like me — the baby boomers. Although that might not seem like such a big deal to you — after all, it's traditionally been incumbent upon succeeding generations to fund health care and the other social services needs of their parents through taxes — the numbers tell a different story.

A 2012 study by J.C. Herbert Emery, David Still, and Thomas Cottrell shows just how impossible a task we're setting for our young people. The study calculates the average taxes paid for health care services over a lifetime for a number of different age groups and compares that number to the amount of health care services used. For Canadians born between 1958 and 1967, we'll eat up over $4,000 more in services than we will have paid for in taxes. But the news gets worse. Those born between 1998 and 2007 will be required to pay over $18,000 more in taxes for health care than they'll use themselves. Those born between 2008 and 2017 will be asked to pay over $27,000. Even more frightening is this statistic: peak taxes for Canadians born after 1988 are projected to be twice as high as peak taxes paid by the oldest of the baby boomers. Still think Canada's health care system is sustainable? Really? Then think about this. If we don't soon get serious and change the way we fund medicare, Canada will be left with no choice but to declare bankruptcy because health care costs are rising much,

much faster than revenues taken in by any of our governments — be they federal, provincial, or territorial.

Let's look at the province of Ontario, as an example. In a five-year period, between 1997–98 and 2002–3, government spending on health care increased by 42 percent, while government revenue increased by only 31 percent. Starting to get scared yet? Listen to this. Prior to 1994–95, the Government of Ontario was spending approximately 32 percent of its annual budget on providing health care services. By 2003–4, health care was eating up almost 40 percent of the budget. Today, in 2019, a whopping 46 percent of the province's budget goes to fund health care. By 2030, experts estimate that, without major changes, health care costs will consume an eye-popping 80 percent of Ontario's budget.

That's crazy.

What's Stopping Us from Doing So?

Those against user fees and co-payments make the argument, more often than not, that forcing patients to pay *extra* for health care is a bad idea because it benefits the well off at the expense of the poor. This is known as the "fairness" argument. It goes something like this. While those opposed to the idea acknowledge that user fees and co-payments would raise more money that could be used to fund our health care system, we must first stop and consider whose pockets these funds would be coming out of. It's an undisputable fact, so the argument goes, that poverty and health are closely linked and that poverty is one of the main causes of poor health outcomes. By shifting some of the burden of paying for medicare from the rich and healthy to the poor and sick, we'd be giving an unfair advantage to some while disadvantaging others.

Further, although user fees and co-payments might well discourage those seeking care unnecessarily, research shows that in many cases they also discourage *necessary* care, as well — especially among the poor. Those making this argument quickly point toward Quebec, where as a result of a cost-sharing plan designed to lower the out-of-control costs of making prescriptions available to its citizens, there was a noticeable reduction in the use of both less essential and essential drugs, which had the unintended consequence of increasing visits to the province's emergency departments. Still other studies show that while 10 percent of Canadians who're prescribed medicine by their family doctors don't bother to fill those prescriptions because of user fees and co-payments, that number rose to over 35 percent among those with low incomes and no insurance.

Then there's the argument that as a result of discouraging the poor and the most vulnerable members of society from seeking care — whether deemed necessary or unnecessary — by forcing them to first pay a "penalty" for seeking help, we might actually be adding to the costs inherent in running our health care system in the long run by creating a situation where those we discouraged from accessing the system are left with no choice but to seek out much more costly treatments down the road as a result of not having been diagnosed and treated earlier.

It's a legitimate argument and highlights a problem we'd need to address if we, as a society, wish to go in the direction I'm proposing. Fortunately, other countries like France, Sweden, and Switzerland have already come up with the solution for us.

Children and those with low incomes in France are exempt from paying co-payments and user fees. In Sweden, the government has placed a ceiling on out-of-pocket payments that caps the amount of money an individual can be charged for accessing health care services. Switzerland takes this concept even further by exempting prenatal and other preventative services from deductibles, user fees, and co-payments.

As a result of injecting fresh funding into our health care system via user fees and co-payments, and allowing more and more freedom of choice for those who are able to take advantage of such things as medical savings accounts, I believe we can actually improve the health care experience in Canada for both the middle class and those not as fortunate. Remember, when you allow private money to mingle with public funds, you're not only providing significant relief to our collective budgetary woes — after all, who wants to see any of our provinces spending 80 percent of their budget on health care within the next ten years — you're also freeing up resources, reducing wait times, and making it possible to treat all patients, no matter where they stand on the socio-economic scale, in a much more timely manner.

Who could possibly have a problem with that?

9. Allow Canadians to Pay for the Services We Want by Introducing a Parallel Private Health Care System and Allowing It to Operate Above Board (the So-Called Hybrid Solution)

Ah, here it is. Finally. At last. The Big One. What some consider to be the third rail of Canadian politics, but what I consider to be the Holy Grail.

It's a dream of mine that one day a politician will emerge from the shadows who has the courage to tell us the truth about our health care system. They will not only be honest about the fact we can't go on like this much longer; they'll also stand up and say that in addition to doing all the things I've already mentioned, Canada must grow up and become an adult and embrace the hybrid solution.

Now, I know some of you will balk at this point and say, "Why should we support a second tier of health care when it will only benefit the rich?" To which I would respond, "The rich don't need a second tier. They already have one. It's called America." The middle class, however — we're the ones who are suffering as a result of this misguided ideal of enforced mediocrity that says, "Everyone must be treated the same, no matter how bad the system gets, or how necessary it is to ration health care."

To the defenders of the status quo, I say, "Be careful what you wish for. You just might get it." To everyone else, my message is simple: when it comes to reforming medicare and reinventing Canada's health care system, we have nothing to lose and everything to gain.

How Might We?

As previously mentioned, back in the late 1990s, when I was still with the Ontario Medical Association, I took a group of about half a dozen doctors — as well as an equal number of OMA staff — to Washington, D.C., where we attended a campaign school organized by the Campaigns & Elections group. At one of the sessions, a presenter told us he was going to teach us to "think outside the box." He made a square using four dots, and then invited us to connect all four dots using *only* three straight lines, ending at the starting point. Most people gave up after about two or three minutes, many saying it was impossible. The answer to this puzzle, for those of you who don't know, is to start with the dot in the upper left-hand corner, and then draw the lines *through* the dots on the top right and lower left and out the other side, so that instead of drawing a box, which can easily be done with *four* straight lines, you end up with a triangle in which all four dots are connected by three straight lines.

Thinking *outside* the box. It's an important lesson I've never forgotten. One those in charge, sadly, seem incapable of learning.

Take health care, for example. With the clock ticking on Canada's 2004 Health Care Accord, Canada's premiers and territorial leaders called on the federal government to increase its health care contribution from 20 to 25 percent. The feds, for their part, were willing to take a look at pouring more money into that vast pit of health care spending but only if the provinces and territories agreed to allow the federal government to "target" where those monies would be spent. "No way," said the premiers. "You don't have the right to interfere with how we spend your health care transfers. The provinces know best and won't be dictated to by anyone." If all this sounds like a bunch of lawyers arguing about semantics, you're right. The problem, to my way of thinking, isn't that we're not throwing enough public money at health care. The real issue is, we, as a country, have allowed ourselves to be boxed in by special interest groups — so much so that today, in 2019, we can't seem to think straight at all.

Don't believe me? Take a look at what's been going on in Ontario. In the summer of 2016, the ministry of health and long-term care and the Ontario Medical Association announced they had reached a deal that would "modernize" (read "cut") the fee schedule, as well as offering up "incentives" (read "bribes") to doctors if they'd help the government identify areas where they could trim $200 million from the health care budget over the following two years — just in time for the 2018 provincial election. Instead of having the courage to come out and admit Ontario's health care system is unsustainable, the Government of Ontario enlisted the help of the OMA to try to convince (read "con") doctors and their patients into believing they had the cure for what ails our health care system — if only the feds up in Ottawa would write them a big enough cheque.

If our elected officials had even one iota of courage, they'd be honest with us and admit the status quo is no longer an option. As I mentioned earlier, should those who have the most to gain by perpetrating this lie continue to play this game, then health care spending will likely eat up 80 percent of our provincial budgets by 2030. This is why we need to start thinking outside the box and why Canada needs a "hybrid" health care system *now*. Remember, even Tommy Douglas was in favour of Canadians paying out of their own pockets as a way of taking pressure off the system. How we ever allowed our health cards to be hijacked by spineless politicians and civil servants and turned into a credit card with no limit is one of those mysteries even Sherlock Holmes wouldn't be able to solve. We can only hope that somewhere, someday, they'll all be forced to swallow some truth serum and admit they've been trying to get us to drink the Kool-Aid all these years.

Why Would We Want To?

Dr. Brian Day, a Canadian physician who founded the Cambie Surgery Centre, a for-profit clinic in Vancouver, in 1995, and a former president of the Canadian Medical Association, is perhaps our country's leading advocate for the reform of Canada's health care system. He launched his Charter challenge ten years ago, after the Supreme Court of Canada ruled that the rights of Quebec residents had been violated by laws that forced citizens to sit on wait-lists while denying them the right to access care outside our publicly funded system. Should this Charter challenge be successful, it'll allow *all* Canadians to exercise rights similar to those available to citizens in other countries. In the autumn of 2016, I had the honour of sitting down with Dr. Day to discuss his Charter challenge against the British Columbia government. We also talked about why Canada's health care system is failing patients and what can be done about it.

> **Q.** You initiated your Charter challenge in January of 2009. Why has it taken so long to get this important issue before a judge?
>
> **A.** The B.C. government has repeatedly stalled. I believe this was in the hope they might force us to abandon the case because of the high cost of litigation. Last year, for instance, just weeks before the trial was to finally begin, the government announced they had discovered 300,000 documents they'd neglected to disclose as required by law. This resulted in a six-month delay. The most recent delay was simply an admission that they needed more time. Wait-lists for access to care and justice are, we have found, both unacceptably long.

Q. Now that it's finally arrived, are you looking forward to your day in court?

A. Absolutely. It's important to recognize the plaintiffs in this case included not only our clinic but six patients who'd suffered at the hands of government failings on access to care. Regrettably, two of the adult cancer sufferers have died during the delay. We were also anxious to emphasize the plight of children on wait-lists, so three children joined us as plaintiffs. The patient plaintiffs in our case represent just six of an estimated two million Canadians who're waiting for care.

Q. What, exactly, is the crux of your argument?

A. Simple. If the government promises necessary care and then fails to deliver it in a timely manner, do they have the right to prevent a citizen from accessing that care independently? Interestingly, those injured at work, RCMP officers, members of the Canadian Armed Forces, and federal prisoners have that right. No country on earth — other than Canada — has such draconian legislation, which forces its citizens to suffer, and even die, on wait-lists. We believe that ordinary Canadians shouldn't have less rights than those who're in jail.

Q. So how is your case different from the Chaoulli case that was successfully argued before the Supreme Court of Canada by Dr. Jacques Chaoulli in 2005?

A. As you state, the Supreme Court of Canada already ruled that residents of Quebec have the right to access private insurance under the Quebec Charter. All seven judges in Chaoulli agreed that patients in Canada were suffering and sometimes dying on wait-lists. We're asking that citizens outside of Quebec have similar protection under the Canadian Charter of Rights and Freedoms. The B.C. and federal governments will be arguing that other Canadians don't deserve similar rights.

Q. If you're successful, and win your Charter challenge, do you think the judge's decision will finally open the door to a hybrid health care system, Canada-wide, by 2020?

A. Even before then. We believe companies that currently offer private medical insurance for such services as prescription drugs, physiotherapy, dentistry, and ambulances, etc. — which are excluded from medicare because they're inaccurately and arbitrarily labelled by civil servants as not being "medically necessary" — will quickly offer full supplemental coverage for all services under their plans. Most Canadians will likely be covered through their employment benefits.

Q. Do Canadians have anything to be afraid of should our country finally, as just about every other country in the world has done, allow a parallel private system to operate alongside — and fully above board with — our public system?

A. On the contrary, we'll see the public system evolve for the better. Public systems in other developed countries collaborate and integrate closely with the private sector in hybrid systems. Wait-lists are non-existent or extremely short in those countries and most spend less on health care than we do.

Q. So, if we have nothing to fear, and our current system is clearly unsustainable, why do you think the vast majority of politicians and union leaders are so in favour of protecting the status quo? Are they simply misguided or do they have an ulterior motive?

A. The public-sector union leadership is afraid of competing with the private sector. The paradox, curiously, is that the most common demographic of a patient treated at private clinics like Cambie Surgery Centre is that of a unionized worker. Most politicians — even those who might deny it publicly — and the majority of the public support our case and want us to win. Competition and choice are not considerations our opponents, such as the union-funded, so-called "health coalitions" and the Canadian Doctors for Medicare group, believe should be offered to Canadians. Strangely, but not surprisingly, those who support a public monopoly, including the groups referenced above, have used services like ours for themselves. Patients treated at our private clinics include leaders from the very groups that're going to court to make sure others can't receive the same benefits they've enjoyed. Hypocrisy reigns supreme.

Q. How do you think Tommy Douglas would view the state of our country's health care system in 2016?

A. I believe that Douglas wouldn't be happy with the current state of affairs, where statistics show the lowest socio-economic groups in Canada have the worst access and suffer the worst health outcomes. This is the opposite of what Douglas' plan was initially intended to do.

Needless to say, this could turn out to be one of the most historic and significant Charter challenges in our nation's history. As Dr. Day has stated elsewhere, it all comes down to the following three questions:

1. Should Canadians in one part of the country — say, British Columbia or Ontario — be forced to suffer on a wait-list, while citizens in another part of the country — say, Quebec — are allowed to purchase and pay for health care services out of their own pockets as a result of the Chaoulli decision?
2. Is it fair that patients whose health care is being covered by some other group — say, workers' compensation, the RCMP, or the armed forces, to mention nothing of those in prison — have superior access to care than the rest of us?
3. Is access to a wait-list really the same thing as access to care?

Once Dr. Day wins his case — and believe me, he will win, of that there is no doubt — I imagine all this will be headed for Ottawa, where the Supreme Court of Canada will hear the same arguments put forth once again. When Dr. Day wins *that* case — and he will — then finally we'll be able to actually do something about fixing our health care system. It may take five years, it may take ten years. But mark my words, the day will come when mediocre is no longer just a synonym for medicare, and we'll have a system we can all truly be proud of.

What's Stopping Us from Doing So?

So, what's stopping us from allowing Canadians to pay for the services we want by introducing a parallel private health care system? In a word: fear. Fear of the unknown. Fear that the less fortunate might be left behind. Fear that so many of our fellow citizens might abandon our public health care system for the private one that our public system might worsen and fall apart. Fear of change. Fear that people like Dr. Jacques Chaoulli and Dr. Brian Day might be right after all. Fear of losing that which makes us Canadian. No doubt about it, people are definitely afraid of embracing the hybrid solution. But should they be?

Let's take a look at each of the above-noted fears and see if we can't put some of this unease to rest.

First and foremost: fear of the unknown. It's human nature that people don't like surprises. I mean, look at how often people stay in bad relationships or re-elect bad governments. "Better the Devil you know," people are wont to say, "than the Devil you don't know." It's ludicrous, of course. Propping up a health care system that's unsustainable and, frankly, broken, while refusing to take a serious look at innovation is not, in my opinion, a recipe for success. It's a recipe for disaster. And yet, time and time again, Canadians embrace the status quo because, bad as things are, at least with our public health care system, you know what you're getting. As I've said elsewhere, when we're talking about our health care system, mediocrity is nothing to shout about. Small wonder Canada has fallen so far down the ladder when it comes to ranking health care systems. Medicare equals mediocre — it's that simple.

Fear that the less fortunate might be left behind. Every time I hear critics of hybrid health care talk about this, I have to laugh. No one is talking about improving the health care experience for the middle class at the expense of the poor and disadvantaged. In fact, it's to everyone's advantage to ensure those at the bottom of the socio-economic scale are well provided for. This tired old canard goes hand in hand with the next fear: fear that so many Canadians might abandon our public health care system for the private one that our public system might worsen and fall apart. There are all kinds of checks and balances we can incorporate into a new made-in-Canada hybrid system — such as legislating a set number of hours a physician must work every month in the public system before switching over and seeing patients in the private one — that there's no way our current health care system will collapse as a result of the introduction of a private system.

The last three things Canadians say they're afraid of — fear of change, fear that people like Dr. Jacques Chaoulli and Dr. Brian Day might be right after all, and fear of losing that which makes us Canadian — are equally silly. Change is good — even if precipitated by a crisis. As I like to tell my clients, a crisis is just an opportunity in disguise. The train wreck that is our health care system presents us with an opportunity to do something truly amazing. But only if we have the courage and wisdom to take that first step. As for Drs. Chaoulli and Day being right … so what? Someone had to climb Mount Everest or land on the moon first. Instead of vilifying these two great Canadian heroes, we should be celebrating them every bit as much as the pro-medicare side celebrates Tommy Douglas.

The last — and, quite possibly, most irrational — fear is that allowing Canadians to pay for the services we want and introducing a parallel private health care system will result in the loss of something that makes us Canadian. In fact, if anything, allowing for freedom and choice — last time I looked — is the most Canadian of Canadian values. Acting like a fascist, on the other hand, isn't something that should be tolerated here in Canada — either by our government or those who think nothing of lying to us.

10. Fund It or Free It

Many years ago, when I was still with the Ontario Medical Association, those of us who wanted to see a hybrid health care system had an expression we liked to toss around. Especially when negotiations with the government of the day had gone off the rails. That expression was: "Fund it or free it." Or, to put it another way, if there wasn't enough money to adequately pay for our publicly funded health care system, then we should be open to looking at new ways of funding it.

But instead of doing something that made sense, health minister after health minister would bash doctors and the doctors would fight back — albeit not particularly effectively. In the end, the two sides would reach an agreement that was "fair and reasonable," totally ignoring all the evidence that medicare as it stood was unsustainable.

Ask Canadians and they'll tell you, not surprisingly, they want as much health care as the government is willing to give them. But they don't want to pay anything for it. And like the father who just can't say "no" to his child, our elected officials have continued to put it all on our collective credit card year after year. Now, the bill is due.

Unless this generation thinks it's all right to stick the next several generations with this expense, we really need to get serious about what we're doing here when it comes to funding medicare.

Yes, our health care system is broken. Although I believe it's not too late to fix it, we urgently need to take the politics and rhetoric out of the equation and try a little straight talk instead. For unless we act now, we'll end up with the very thing all of us agree that we don't want — namely, a U.S.-style, two-tier health care system.

How Might We?

Fund it or free it. Five simple words. Straightforward, uncomplicated, and to the point. So why do so many people have such a hard time with the concept? Again, I have a theory. When you cut through all the clutter, it all comes down to one thing: perception. Our leaders, at least those currently heading up governments here in Canada, don't want to be seen as the ones who allowed our health care system to fail so badly they were left with no choice but to finally embrace the hybrid solution. Like in the game hot potato, those in charge keep passing the buck. Take the Province of Ontario, for instance. As previously mentioned, it's my understanding that the Ontario government has funded dozens of studies and papers, whose only purpose is to provide a blueprint for getting out of this mess. Basically, they want to be able to find a way to allow a parallel private health care system without having to wear it and ultimately take the blame for it. Such a fear is unfounded, though. I believe that the vast majority of voters would not see such a change as a negative thing. In fact, I think the vast majority would actually support a political party that had the guts to admit the obvious and show a little leadership on the issue.

But, as everyone knows, that is in short supply these days.

These frightened little mice who govern us need not be afraid, however, for I suspect that sooner or later our courts will make the decisions for them. We've already seen the kind of changes the Supreme Court of Canada has brought about in Quebec as a result of the Chaoulli decision. We're likely to see something similar in British Columbia, once the courts make their final ruling on Dr. Day's Charter challenge. It's only a matter of time before common sense prevails and our elected officials are forced to do the right thing and move Canada away from a single-payer system and into the twenty-first century. Until that happens, though, I'm afraid more of our fellow citizens are going to have to suffer on wait-lists and even die waiting for treatment.

It doesn't have to be that way.

The ten solutions I've put forth, as I've taken great pains to point out, are, while controversial, nonetheless very doable. Politicians *can* stop lying to us. They *can* put patients first and ideology second. It *is* possible for us to revise the Canada Health Act so that "quality" becomes the sixth principle. We *can* combine all of Canada's provincial and territorial health ministries into one federal super ministry with one health minister. Government *has* the wherewithal to stop focusing on illness and instead figure out how to keep us healthy. There *is* no reason we can't open the door to medical tourism. Canada *has* the resources, right here, right now, to invest heavily in long-term care. With the wave of a wand, government *can* bring back co-payments and user fees and introduce tax-free medical savings accounts. They *can* allow Canadians to pay for the services we want by introducing a parallel private health care system, the so-called hybrid solution, and allowing it to operate above board. And, of course, those in charge *are* perfectly capable of funding our health care system or freeing it.

So why don't they?

As I stated earlier, it all comes down to perception. In politics, perception is not only more important that reality, most will tell you that perception *is* reality. If I, as leader of X Party, can convince the voters that you, as leader of Y Party, have a hidden agenda to put medicare, as we know it, at risk by allowing change and innovation, thereby putting Canada on the slippery slope toward having a two-tier health care system, then I just might be able to demonize you enough in the minds of the electorate to win the next election. Unless you and your party are able to convince the voters that it is, in fact, *I* who have the hidden agenda, and that I'll be the one who paves the way for the privatization of Canada's health care system by delisting services and making other changes to the fee schedule. And on and on and on. It's sick, it's perverse, it's disgusting. But it's the way the health care debate has been framed in our country for the past sixty years.

Why Would We Want To?

Tell me if you think I'm nuts. But here's what I envision.

We put together a public relations campaign. We build a website. We create some ads and print up a bunch of pamphlets. We hand out buttons that say, "Fund it or free it." We hold a media conference. We do five, ten, fifteen, twenty interviews on TV and radio. We write op-eds for news-papers, telling our side of the story. "Canada's health care system, as it's currently configured, is unsustainable. The status quo is getting in the way of innovation. We need a hybrid system and we need it now. Tomorrow will be too late." We set up a bunch of town hall meetings. We hold a rally on Parliament Hill. We do what I tell all of my clients they must do in order to successfully change minds and win the day.

Educate. Motivate. Activate.

We do all these things … and then we do them again. Over and over and over. They say someone has to hear a message six times, delivered three different ways, before it starts to sink in. I call this the "six-and-three rule." So, we do this. Until finally, one by one, city by city, town by town, prov-ince by province, territory by territory, we get as many people as possible on board in order to finally fix our country's health care system once and for all. I could die happy then, knowing in my heart of hearts I'd not only done all I could but had actually succeeded in reinventing Canada's health care system along with you and the rest of our fellow citizens.

Will such a campaign succeed? If it does, it won't be because there wasn't any opposition. For as soon as we go public, the other side will rear its ugly head and begin barking as loud as they possibly can.

"If you allow private health care into Canada, we'll lose the essence of what our country is all about."

"Private health care isn't about patient care. Not really. It's about allowing a doctor to charge whatever he or she wants to charge for a service that's already covered by medicare while billing both the public and private systems."

"If we loosen the rules and allow private medicine to become a part of our system, then doctors will be in a position to help those who're in pain and vulnerable to jump the queue in order to receive treatment at a private facility much faster than they normally would at a public one. This wouldn't be right."

"Admittedly, Canada's health care system isn't without its challenges. But allowing a private system to operate right alongside our public one … well, that cure would be even worse than the disease. We simply can't allow such a thing here in Canada."

Yes, our battle won't be an easy one. Things are bound to turn nasty along the way. Forget about "lies, damned lies, and statistics." There's so much at stake here the other side will stop at nothing to get their way. Fortunately, we have a secret weapon: the truth.

If you find yourself often shaking your head listening to what our elected officials have to say, it just might be because what they're telling us has no basis in fact. The truth is Canada's health care system needs a major overhaul. A tweak here and a tweak there simply isn't going to cut it anymore. Neither is dumping wheelbarrows full of cash into the bottomless pit that is medicare. Remember, Paul Martin's fix for a generation lasted only ten years and, when all was said and done, fixed nothing. No, we don't need any more quick fixes. What we really require is a commitment from those whose responsibility it is to do something about the mess we find ourselves in. Needless to say, finding a solution to this problem will take a whole lot more than pretty words and empty promises. It'll take intestinal fortitude, a vision that Canadians can get behind, and a willingness to see it through.

All of which invites the question: "If they can't or won't fund it, will they have the courage to free it?"

What's Stopping Us from Doing So?

Sometimes, when I lie in bed at night, I think about my parents and my brothers, the one who's still here and the one who isn't, and wonder if any of this is worth it. My mother used to tell my brothers and me that we didn't have the sense "God gave a goose" whenever we'd done something particularly dumb, like breaking a window playing hockey on the backyard rink or putting out the knees in a new pair of pants playing a board game on the cement floor in the basement. If she were still alive, if our health care system hadn't killed her a few years ago, I wonder what my mother would make of those in charge of Canada's health care system.

Or perhaps my dad. He'd have had something to say for sure. He had to quit school and get a job as a grocery boy to help his family make it through the Great Depression, and then went off to fight in the Second World War, before coming home in 1945 and spending the next thirty-plus years climbing poles in all kinds of weather as a Bell Telephone lineman until he turned sixty. Well, I can't help thinking my dad would've been none too impressed with this lot. Whenever I'd bring some injustice, perceived or otherwise, to his attention as a young boy and ask him for his thoughts on the matter, my father would inevitably say something like, "It all depends on whose ox is being gored." On those rare occasions when a politician actually said something that made sense, my dad would reply with: "There's more truth than poetry in that statement."

From my unique vantage point, as a temp working in various ministries, as a political staffer, as a lobbyist for Ontario's doctors, and as a consultant for a number of health care clients, I've been afforded the unique opportunity over the past thirty years or so to witness both the best and worst of health care in Canada. Those frontline providers of care — doctors, nurses, pharmacists, and other health care professionals too numerous to list — are the *real* heroes, in my way of thinking. Day after day, they selflessly make sacrifice after sacrifice, saving lives and helping patients recover from injury and illness with nary a thought for their own safety or mental health. And while it'd be way too simplistic to paint every elected official and every civil servant as a villain, the fact remains those who aren't providing frontline care, those who're, for the most part, working behind the scenes, hidden away, completely anonymous, are the ones who're responsible for the mess we're in. They're the ones who've come up with what I like to call "schemes and dreams," the ones who seem to have taken the anti-Hippocratic oath. Instead of "doing no harm," these people appear to be out to do as much harm as possible. The Patients First Act. The Protecting Patients Act. If only.

• • •

Finally, before we part ways, let me leave you with a story about the wise old man who was said to be able to answer any question — a story that seems particularly relevant in light of the journey we've just taken together.

A young boy thought he could trick the sage, so he caught a bird and took it to him. "Tell me, is the bird in my hands dead or alive?"

The wise old man replied, "If I say the bird is alive, you'll close your hands and crush it to death. If, on the other hand, I say the bird is dead, you'll open your hands and it'll fly away."

He paused for a bit and then smiled. "The answer," he said, "is in your hands."

The Big Fix

Ten things those in charge could do tomorrow to reinvent and ultimately fix Canada's health care system:

1. Stop lying to us.
2. Put patients first, ideology second.
3. Revise the Canada Health Act so that "quality" becomes the sixth principle.
4. Combine all of Canada's provincial and territorial health ministries into one federal "super ministry" with one health minister.
5. Stop focusing on illness and figure out how to keep us healthy instead.
6. Open the door to "medical tourism."
7. Invest heavily in long-term care — or be prepared to face the consequences.
8. Bring back co-payments and user fees and introduce tax-free medical savings accounts.
9. Allow Canadians to pay for the services we want by introducing a parallel private health care system, and allow it to operate above board (the so-called hybrid solution).
10. Fund it or free it.

CODA

"THAT'S ALL, FOLKS!"

Our journey is almost done. We have travelled many miles together, you and I, and seen many things. We have explored the myriad of myths that have grown up around our health care system in much the same way some people explore caves. We have studied the history of medicare in this country in hopes of not repeating the mistakes of the past. Finally, we have carefully examined the schemes and dreams of others, who failed to save Canada's health care system not because they were bad people but because they lacked the vision and courage to think outside the box and reach for the stars.

Yes, our journey is nearly complete. But I still have a few more things to say.

Let's start by addressing the elephant in the room. Embracing the hybrid solution when it comes to health care doesn't make you a traitor. Nor does it mean you're in favour of adopting a U.S.-style, two-tier health care system. I have to laugh every time one of my critics uses this line of reasoning to attack me. Why on earth would anyone push for bringing America's failed ideas to Canada when study after study shows that what our neighbours to the south have is so much worse than our system?

I'm also amused by the other argument that some like to throw at people like Dr. Brian Day and me — that we have a hidden agenda and secretly want to do away with Canada's public health care system and replace it with a private one. Not once, not one single time, has anyone in favour of reinventing our health care system ever suggested it would be a good idea to replace our public system with a private system. Not once. And yet, time and time again, those defenders of the status quo throw themselves into battle, waving the flag and saying things like, "We must defend medicare against those who would do it harm!" What a bunch of baloney. I mean, if Dr. Day and I really did want to replace medicare in Canada with a private health care system, then all we'd have to do is what all these others are doing. For as I've said elsewhere and often, the best way to ensure we end up with a system like they currently have in America is to do nothing. For burying your head in the sand and pretending Canada's health care system is the best in the world and sustainable is a surefire way to guarantee its demise.

Don't believe me? Then ask yourself a simple question: "If Canada's health care system is so good, so worth fighting for and preserving, then why hasn't anyone else copied what we're doing?" The answer, my friend, is simple. Our system sucks. While we've been standing around for the past fifty-plus years, admiring our collective navels, everyone else has been embracing not the status quo but change. Real change. Real innovation. Real solutions for an ever-evolving world.

What Tommy Douglas came up with in the late 1940s was fine for back then. What Justice Emmett Hall recommended in the mid-1960s did the trick back in the day. What Monique Bégin envisioned in 1983 was what was thought to be necessary thirty-six years ago. Unfortunately, time, as we all know, doesn't stand still. In order to be great, we have to innovate. As we have seen, those in charge are afraid of change. Very afraid. "It's the third rail of Canadian politics," they say. "Only a fool would dare to suggest introducing a parallel private health care system. Voters would toss you out in a heartbeat if you dared to mess with medicare. It may not be perfect," they continue, "but it's better than all the alternatives." This way of thinking is why, election after election, we never talk about health care, we never have a meaningful debate about what's right with our system and what's wrong and what's so badly in need of fixing.

Too bad. Because the fact is, if our leaders actually had any *cojones* at all, they'd come clean and admit the truth, that Canada's health care system is unsustainable; is badly in need of significant, long-lasting change and not just tweaking; and that we can't afford to go on pretending everything is all right when it obviously isn't. Oh, and one other thing. It's my belief that if someone *did* emerge and showed the courage to admit these things and embrace the hybrid solution, their party would win a massive majority when the next election rolled around.

Seriously.

This is why I decided to write a book and embark on this journey with you. The kinds of changes I've been talking about will happen only if we take charge and start showing our leaders how to lead. In this day and age, most of them prefer to lead from the middle. That's not leading, it's *following*. History tells us that a real leader *listens* first, then *acts*. Regrettably, those currently in power like to impose their will on us, without bothering to listen. And so long as the polls tell them what to do, what's safe and what's palatable, they'll continue to feed us, the voters, the bland, tasteless pablum they've been forcing down our throats for decades. But it doesn't have to be that way. We can do something about this. We can effect change. If, and only if, we're willing to stand up for ourselves. Remember, *we*, not politicians, and most surely not the civil service, own Canada's health care system. We pay for it out of our taxes and we're the ones who suffer when health care is rationed and we're forced to wait and wait and wait.

A Canadian health care revolution: it's what we need and what we want.

How Might We Fix Canada's Health Care System (and Why Would We Want To)?

Albert Einstein defined insanity as doing the same thing over and over again and expecting different results. I can't think of a better way to describe the approach taken by elected officials and civil servants when it comes to reforming Canada's health care system. It *is* pure insanity, watching prime ministers, premiers, and health ministers, year after year, do what I like to call "the health care cha-cha-cha" — seemingly moving forward, backward, and sideways all at the same time. It would be funny if it weren't so painful to watch. Honestly, it's astonishing to see the lengths to which governments will go to convince us they have things under control when clearly they don't. They call media conferences. They make announcements. They organize photo ops, complete with the obligatory selfie. Then they do it all over again, re-announcing what they announced six months ago. It reminds me of someone playing Russian roulette. "Around and around she goes, where she stops nobody knows" — until the gun does not just click and someone gets their head blown off. Which, not surprisingly, is usually one of us.

So, how *do* we fix Canada's health care system? Even more importantly, why would we want to? Well, for one thing, people might start by admitting it's broken and needs fixing. It would also be useful if we were a little more adept at identifying the problem instead of always allowing ourselves to be distracted by stuff that, at the end of the day, doesn't add up to a hill of beans. As former Ontario health minister Elizabeth Witmer told George Smitherman after he appeared before the legislative committee looking into the Commitment to the Future of Medicare Act back in 2004, the reason people were paying money to jump the queue was because they were waiting too long for treatment. Now, someone with even one iota of common sense would conclude that something needed to be done about wait times. Those in charge, however, instead decided what was really needed was something that could measure how long a patient would typically have to wait for a specific procedure. Hence the birth of the wait-list website.

Pure madness, right?

Even crazier are some of the ideas being put forth by Dr. Danielle Martin and the Canadian Doctors for Medicare group. They claim that Canada's health care system is fine just as it is. All it needs are a few *tweaks* here and there, and a fresh infusion of cash. Lots and lots of cash. For example, let's fund a national pharmacare program. And while we're at it, how about a guaranteed minimum income for those at the bottom of the socio-economic spectrum? Oh, and don't forget to tax the living daylights out of doctors. They make too much money anyway and should be grateful for having the privilege of dealing with the mess that is medicare.

We don't need this kind of thinking. And we certainly don't need these kinds of solutions. Not unless you're looking to bankrupt the country, or have the government spend every nickel and dime they take from taxpayers on health care. Because if you do that, as I said before, then you'll be left with no choice but to privatize our education system and turn every road into a toll road. Something I don't think most Canadians would be onside with. No, what we really need is a *strategy* — call it a road map or a blue-print, I really don't care — one that lays out a plan in a logical manner and addresses the real problems Canada's health care system faces while offering up real solutions. No more health care cha-cha-cha. No more spending like drunken sailors. And for God's sake, no more wrapping oneself in the flag of patriotism.

"Fund it or free it." It's more than a slogan. It's a philosophy. And a basic human right. After all, if we can spend money on cigarettes and booze — things we know can do us harm — then why on earth are we prohibited from spending money on health care? If it's perfectly fine for someone to put aside money in order to buy a big-screen television or save up for a winter vacation in the Caribbean, then what's wrong with setting up a medical savings account and squirrelling money away for a future medical procedure or health care catastrophe? Medicare needn't be mediocre. As Oscar Wilde once famously put it, "We are all in the gutter, but some of us are looking at the stars." Dare to dream and you just might be surprised to discover that when it comes to health care in this country, we can do better. A whole lot better. But only if we stand up for ourselves.

What's Stopping Us from Doing So?

One of the biggest impediments to progress, I believe, is this obsession that's developed over the past few years with metrics. "If you can't measure it," these techno wizards like to say, "you can't manage it." It's a pithy phrase that sounds good, and makes for a memorable sound bite, but it's one that's ultimately meaningless. Case in point: when the Ontario government announced it was launching a series of primary care reform pilot projects in the early 2000s, they made a big deal about how they were going to closely monitor everything so we could see for ourselves whether moving away from paying doctors on a fee-for-service basis was a good thing or a bad thing. Well, the pilots went ahead, the doctors and patients did their thing, and the consultants — who were not cheap, by the way — made their measurements and crunched the numbers and cashed their cheques.

And then ... nothing.

The government didn't release the results to the public. Instead, they suppressed the consultants' reports and announced the pilots had been so successful the province was going to get behind primary care reform in a big way. Thus began the whole alphabet soup of primary care health models — FHGs, FHNs, FHOs, FHTs. Great stuff, right? Only, as it turned out, Ontario soon discovered just how costly primary care reform truly was. After a decade or so of paying doctors *not* to see patients or spend money on tests and other exploratory interventions, the government decided they couldn't afford the program. Ironically, it turned out that much maligned fee-for-service was actually a more economical way to pay doctors in spite of everything. Something I suspect those original consultant reports probably showed.

The biggest impediment to creating a hybrid health care system in Canada, though, is without a doubt the silliest. "If we allow a second tier of health care," the argument goes, "it will only benefit the rich." Every time I hear this, I have to shake my head. It's so ludicrous. Remember, the rich don't need a second tier of health care. They already have it. It's called the United States. If the fabulously well-to-do need treatment and need it now, they simply hop on a plane and go to the MD Anderson Cancer Center in Texas or the Mayo Clinic in Minnesota or one of any number of private clinics down south.

The people who would benefit most from a parallel private health care system, interestingly enough, are you and me — the middle class. The boomers and zoomers. We're the ones who'd be most likely to take advantage of a hybrid system if we had one. And, ultimately, we're the ones that are going to drive this issue, because there's no way any of us are going to put up with waiting a ridiculous amount of time for knee and hip replacements or cataract surgery. Our generation is both active and proactive — it's unlikely we'd allow some mealy-mouthed politician to tell us we can't make our way to the front of the line to get back on the golf course or tennis court as soon as possible.

Of course, the whole debate about two-tier health care in Canada is something of a joke anyway. We have so many tiers, it's frankly hard to keep track. There's the workers' compensation tier. The RCMP and Canadian Forces' tier. The professional athletes' tier. The politicians' tier. The friends of friends' tier. And so on and so forth. Honestly, just having two tiers would be an improvement. But those living in the "Land of Make-Believe" continue to insist we only have one tier of health care in Canada, and probably will until the day they die.

Which brings us to the final reason I wrote this book. After having almost bought the farm a few years ago, I realized just how precious life is and how few years I have left. I like to joke that I've signed up for the Freedom 105 program, that I'll own my own home and be able to retire when I turn 105. But the fact is there are simply not enough hours left on the clock or days in the year for me to accomplish everything I've set out to do. This is why I decided to concentrate on doing one thing and one thing only — fix Canada's health care system before it implodes. And while some people don't like what I have to say, and have gone to great lengths to silence me, the fact remains I'm still standing and still fighting for what I believe in.

That's it. I'm done. I've got nothing more to add. I'm out of here. Or at least I would be if only it wasn't for the look on your face. Because I can tell something's bothering you. And if there are two things I've learned over the years as a lobbyist, they are these: you don't leave money on the table, and you never, ever fail to close the deal. So, let me see if I can answer the question I imagine you're longing to ask. "How do we know this isn't all one big con, and that you're not just spinning us?"

Let me be frank with you. You really don't have any way of knowing whether or not I've been telling the truth all this time or talking out of my hat. Let me just say for the record, however, that everything you've heard come out of my mouth during the time we've spent together on our journey is the truth, the whole truth, and nothing but the *truth*. Although it's true I do have an agenda — *everyone* has an agenda, by the way, even those who say they don't have one — my sole purpose in pointing out what's wrong with our health care system is simply to make it possible for people like us to do something about it.

Still not convinced? If it makes it any easier for you, why not try this? Just say the Devil made me do it. That's why I wrote this book. That's why I've fought so hard against the status quo and all those who keep putting up all kinds of unnecessary roadblocks to impede real reform and innovation. That's why I continue to advocate for a hybrid health care system. All I ask is that you have a little sympathy for the Devil. For while it may be true I'm a hard man to like, and an even harder man to trust, you can't deny my heart's in the right place. In the meantime, if you still believe Canada has the best health care system in the world, that it isn't a bloody mess, and it's not time we do something about it, then what can I say? Just close the book, ignore the evidence, and pretend everything is fine.

But what if I'm right?

⊢━━━▶ ACKNOWLEDGEMENTS ◀━━━⊣

Just as no man is an island, no book or author is an island, either. This book would not exist without the generous support and contributions of the following people …

First and foremost, I need to thank Jim Cooper, my favourite Dutch uncle, who not only taught me everything I know about politics, but who also explained the importance of having a family and why it was maybe time to stop acting like a kid in a candy store and finally settle down.

I'm also most grateful to Dan Rath, who educated me on how the media works, and who made all those trips to Washington, D.C., not only possible but also memorable.

Special shout-out to Jeff Henry, long-time editor of the *Ontario Medical Review*, and my former colleague at the Ontario Medical Association. Jeff was the first person who thought something I wrote might be worth publishing, so I guess we'll have to blame him for this book taking up space on your shelf.

Thanks to Richard Worzel for his friendship over the years and his incredible insights. I'm also indebted to him for helping me understand that the future is now.

To Buzz Hargrove, what can I say? It's been an honour and a privilege to work with you, as well as call you my friend.

Many thanks to Steve Paikin, Gilbert Sharpe, and Jaime Watt. Your contributions to this book and to my life in general have been huge, and I cherish the time we've spent together, either in person or in cyberspace.

Speaking of good friends, I'd also like to thank Ted Woloshyn for all he's done for me. Ted was kind enough to invite me on his show many years ago, thus launching my career in radio. Let's hope he doesn't come to his senses any time soon and realize what a mistake that was.

In a similar vein, let me pay tribute to Charles Adler, who had me on his TV show in 2012 to discuss the need for a hybrid health care system in Canada before any of us were even calling it that.

Thank yous are also due to Dr. Brian Day, Dr. Barry Dworkin, Dr. Merrilee Fullerton, Dr. Bill Hughes, Dr. Akbar Khan, Dr. Ed Klimek, Dr. Robert Kwan, Dr. Douglas Mark, Dr. Keith Meloff, Dr. Charles Shaver, Dr. Michael Thoburn, Dr. John Tracey, and Dr. Shawn Whatley. Canada is lucky to have such wonderful, dedicated doctors, and I'm particularly blessed to call you my friends.

Loving thoughts to Irene Hsu, in memory of her husband, Dr. Anthony Hsu.

My deepest gratitude goes out to my dear friend and colleague Lorraine Weygman, who not only introduced me to Dr. Min Basadur and Simplexity (about which more later), but who also convinced me it's never too late to accomplish your life's work, so long as you remain committed and show up on time every day.

Thank you, thank you, thank you to my editors Dominic Farrell and Jenny McWha, freelance editor Laurie Miller, my publicists Michelle Melski and Tabassum Siddiqui, and all the rest of the gang at Dundurn. You somehow managed to turn the mess of a manuscript I delivered into something resembling a book, and I can't thank you enough.

Kudos to my agent Arnold Gosewich, who took me under his wing and taught me to fly. I don't know where I'd be without him.

Special thanks to Peter Gabany of Limelight Advertising & Design, who made me smile and then captured it on film.

Much love to my mother-in-law, Donna Ellul, for her unwavering support before, during, and after the writing of this book, in addition to all those lovely care packages she keeps sending home with us whenever we go to visit her.

I'm also indebted to the many friends and colleagues who pulled out their chequebooks and supported me financially these past couple of years. Thank you one and all.

Extra special thanks to my mom and dad, John and Shirley Skyvington, who never stopped believing in me. I only wish they were still alive to celebrate this book.

And, of course, I can't forget my brothers, Jim and Brian, who taught me the importance of getting back up and shaking it off no matter how badly it hurt.

Nor can I forget my dogs (Cooper, Jack, Maxwell, Riggs, and Sammy), each of whom has made every day a little bit better just by being a part of my life.

Last but not least, thank you to my lovely wife, Michelle, and our boy, Joshua, who saved my life in more ways than one.

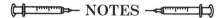 NOTES

Prologue: The Roots of Coincidence

The Roots of Coincidence is the name of a 1972 book by Arthur Koestler, which examines parapsychology, extrasensory perception, and psychokinesis. The musician Sting, who was somewhat enthralled by Koestler, named The Police's final studio album *Synchronicity* as a homage to *The Roots of Coincidence*. "The Roots of Coincidence" is also the name of a song by the Pat Metheny Group, featured on their 1997 album *Imaginary Day*.

The ancient proverb "A journey of a thousand miles begins with a single step" is said to have been first coined by Chinese philosopher Lao Tzu, although it's often incorrectly attributed to Confucius.

For more on Monique Bégin, readers are encouraged to check out her book, *Medicare: Canada's Right to Health* (Ottawa: Optimum, 1988).

Many articles have been written about the 1986 doctors' strike in Ontario, but perhaps the best of the bunch was written by Jim Coyle ("Clashes between governments and doctors have long history"), which appeared in the May 12, 2012, edition of the *Toronto Star*. A worthy companion piece to Jim Coyle's article would be the controversial bestseller written by Dan Rath and Georgette Gagnon, *Not Without Cause: David*

Peterson's Fall From Grace (Toronto: HarperCollins, 1991), which not only goes into quite some detail about the 1986 doctors' strike in Ontario, but also examines the root causes for David Peterson and the Liberals' stunning election loss to Bob Rae and the NDP on September 6, 1990.

The night of the long knives was a purge that took place in Nazi Germany in 1934, when Adolf Hitler ordered a series of executions meant to consolidate his hold on power.

To learn more about the Ontario Medical Association, please visit their website at oma.org. Those looking to better understand medical politics may wish to take out a subscription with the *Medical Post* (canadianhealthcarenetwork.ca). Another excellent source of health care information can be found online at healthydebate.ca.

I'd be remiss if I didn't mention the huge contribution Dr. Min Basadur and his team at Basadur Applied Creativity made to this book. Without Min's remarkable Simplexity thinking system, there's no way I could've organized all my thoughts and ideas and presented them clearly, concisely, and comprehensively. While the conclusions I come to, and the solutions I offer up in Part IV, "The Big Fix," are all my own, the Simplexity system (including the three questions I pose in Part IV: "How might we?"; "Why would we want to?"; and "What's stopping us from doing so?") is all his. I invite you to visit their website at basadur.com and consider taking one of their many marvellous courses.

Part I: Back to the Future

Back to the Future is the name of a 1985 science fiction film directed by Robert Zemeckis. It stars Michael J. Fox as a teenager who accidentally travels back in time to 1955, where he meets his future parents and becomes his mother's romantic interest. The phrase "back to the future" typically refers to something from the past that's been recycled in the present, often being presented as if it were something new.

For those interested in learning more about Dr. Danielle Martin's approach, I highly recommend you read her book, *Better Now: Six Big Ideas to Improve Health Care for All Canadians* (Toronto: Allen Lane, 2017). Although I strongly disagree with her solutions, one can't deny that she's written a thoughtful, important book. Another book readers may wish to take a look at was written by Raisa B. Deber and entitled, *Treating Health Care: How the Canadian System Works and How It Could Work Better* (Toronto: University of Toronto Press, 2017). A professor, she presents an academic's point of view, which stands in stark contrast to what I've presented here in my book.

There've been a number of first-rate books written about Tommy Douglas. Of particular note is one written by Vincent Lam for the Extraordinary Canadians series, entitled simply *Tommy Douglas* (Toronto: Viking, 2011). Two other books well worth checking out were written by Dave Margoshes, *Tommy Douglas: Building the New Society* (Toronto: Dundurn, 1999), and Walter Stewart, *The Life and Political Times of Tommy Douglas* (Toronto: McArthur & Company, 2003). One final book readers may wish to examine was written by Thomas McLeod, entitled *Tommy Douglas: The Road to Jerusalem* (Markham, ON: Fifth House Publishers, 2004).

While researching Tommy Douglas and the 1962 Saskatchewan doctors' strike, I benefitted greatly from reading the following articles: "Tommy Douglas, the pragmatic socialist," by Neil Reynolds, *Globe and Mail*, November 20, 2010; "We should honour Tommy Douglas' vision," by Gregory Marchildon, *National Post*, January 26, 2012; "Reforming Medicare: What would Tommy Douglas do?," by Shaun Francis, *National Post*, June 29, 2012; "The birth of medicare," by Lorne Brown and Doug Taylor, *Canadian Dimension*, July 3, 2012; and "CCF Premier Tommy Douglas changed the face of his adopted country," by Craig Baird, *Regina Leader-Post*, updated June 28, 2017. An essay by Dr. Michael Rachlis ("Completing the Vision: Achieving the Second Stage of Medicare"), which first appeared in September 2007 on the Canadian Centre for Policy Alternatives website, was also helpful.

For those interested in learning more about Justice Emmett Hall, I'd direct your attention to two fine books: *Emmett Hall: Establishment Radical* by Dennis Gruending (Toronto: MacMillan of Canada, 1985) and *Aggressive in Pursuit: The Life of Justice Emmett Hall* by Frederick Vaughan (Toronto: University of Toronto Press, 2004). In addition to these two books, I also found reminisces by former Saskatchewan premiers Allan Blakeney ("The Struggle to Implement Medicare," May 2007) and Roy Romanow ("Medicare and Beyond: A 21st Century Vision," August 2009) to be invaluable in helping to piece together the story of the birth of medicare in Saskatchewan during the Tommy Douglas era. A paper by Dr. Jacalyn Duffin ("The Impact of Single-Payer Health Care on Physician Income in Canada, 1850–2005") was both informative and eye-opening. Lastly, I'd suggest every Canadian read a copy of Justice Hall's final report, which was issued on June 19, 1964 (Volume I), and December 7, 1964 (Volume II). Although copies of the Hall Commission's report can be hard to find, with a little detective work it's possible to find one or both volumes at some public libraries or university libraries.

Strangely, despite the fact Canadians seemingly do nothing but talk about it, no one to date has written a book about the Canada Health Act. Nevertheless, several thoughtful and incisive articles have appeared in the media over the years, including: "At 25, the Canada Health Act deserves better from our leaders," by André Picard, *Globe and Mail*, August 20, 2009; "Save health care: Give the Canada Health Act a sunset clause," by Colin Busby, *National Post*, March 7, 2011; and "Scrap the Canada Health Act," by Dr. Harry Pollett, *Halifax Chronicle Herald*, September 2, 2017. Another solid piece of scholarship I leaned on was written by Brian Lindenberg ("The Canada Health Act: Then, now and in 2014"), which first appeared in March 2012 on the *Benefits Canada* website. I also found an article in the January 15, 1985, edition of the *Canadian Medical Association Journal* ("The provinces and the profession: Assessing the impact of the Canada Health Act") to be most useful in understanding how the medical profession was impacted all across the country by this new piece of legislation.

There are two exceptional books on Mike Harris and the Common Sense Revolution that I'd like to bring your attention to. The first was written by Christina Blizzard, *Right Turn: How the Tories Took Ontario* (Toronto: Dundurn, 1995), while the second was penned by John Ibbitson, *Promised Land: Inside the Mike Harris Revolution* (Toronto: Prentice Hall, 1997). Both are seminal works that go a long way toward helping us understand not only what happened in 1995, when Mike Harris and the PC Party of Ontario went from third place to first in a little over a month, but also why it happened. A third book, which I found totally fascinating, was written by Duncan Sinclair, Mark Rochon, and Peggy Leatt, *Riding the Third Rail: The Story of Ontario's Health Services Restructuring Commission, 1996–2000* (Montreal and Kingston: McGill-Queen's University Press, 2005).

While I was fortunate (or *unfortunate*, depending upon your point of view) to have had a front-row seat during the entire Savings and Restructuring Act debate in 1995–96, a number of wonderful articles by various members of the Queen's Park press gallery helped refresh my memory. However, it was a June 22, 2015, blog post by TVO's Steve Paikin ("The Common Sense Revolution at 20 lives on") that best captured, to my way of thinking, this truly sensitive time in Ontario's history.

In researching the Commitment to the Future of Medicare Act, I spent hours poring through the Ontario Hansard, especially the sections dealing with committee hearings looking into the legislation. If you've never been to Queen's Park and sat in on a committee hearing, do yourself a favour and check it out. Much more than question period, which, after all, is little more than theatre of the absurd on most days, committee hearings are where the actual work gets done and bills become law. While admittedly it's a bit like going to a factory and watching how they make sausages, it's a worthwhile exercise in democracy nonetheless.

Three books proved particularly helpful during the writing of the section exploring the Commitment to the Future of Medicare Act. Two were autobiographies: *Greg Sorbara: The Battlefield of Ontario Politics* (Toronto: Dundurn, 2014) and *Dalton McGuinty: Making a Difference* (Toronto: Dundurn, 2015). A third book, which was written by Daniel Dickin and was most definitely *not* an autobiography, entitled *Liars: The McGuinty-Wynne Record* (Toronto: Freedom Press, 2014), was of great use in helping me keep the Ontario Liberals' many scandals straight.

Part II: "If It's Free, It's for Me"

The first time I heard the phrase "If it's free, it's for me" I just about fell out of my chair. I was sitting in an MPP's office at Queen's Park, along with Dr. Michael Thoburn, executive director of professional services at the Ontario Medical Association, trying to explain the importance of working with doctors instead of against them, when Mike uttered those immortal words.

I found many articles that explained in no uncertain terms why our "free" health care system isn't quite so free after all. Among the best was an article by Brian Lee Crowley ("This report just shredded every myth claiming

Canadian medicare is superior — or fair") that appeared in the July 25, 2017, edition of the *Financial Post,* and another by Bacchus Barua of the Fraser Institute ("How Much 'Free' Health Care Really Costs Canadians") that ran in the October 17, 2014, edition of the *Huffington Post.*

Speaking of the Fraser Institute, readers would be well advised to explore their website at fraserinstitute.org, where you'll find many well-researched articles and studies on the subject of health care. I've relied heavily throughout the book on the fine work of the institute and recommend their organization as a trusted source of information. Another handy depository of health care facts and figures is the Canadian Institute for Health Information (cihi.ca). CIHI's charts and graphics help make the hazy maze of health care statistics easy for anyone to understand.

Perhaps the best place to start any discussion about private health care being the "third rail" of Canadian politics is Jeffrey Simpson's remarkable book, *Chronic Condition: Why Canada's Health Care System Needs to be Dragged into the 21st Century* (Toronto: Allen Lane, 2012). Another fine book that touches on a wide variety of topics, including many that I examine in Part II of my book, is *Matters of Life and Death: Public Health Issues in Canada* (Madeira Park, BC: Douglas & McIntyre, 2017) by André Picard. Although I don't always agree with everything Simpson and Picard say, both are passionate about Canadian health care and truly know their stuff.

In addition to these two books, there's no shortage of articles about health care and the third rail, including a thoughtful piece by Jaime Watt ("It's time to talk about private healthcare"), which ran in the October 23, 2016, edition of the *Toronto Star.* Alastair Rickard's article ("A puzzled Canadian ponders surreal U.S. health-care debate"), which appeared in the September 9, 2009, edition of the *Toronto Star* is also well worth checking out. Going back even further, readers would be well advised to delve into an article by Clifford Kraus ("Canada's Private Clinics Surge as Public System Falters") that ran in the February 28, 2006, edition of the *New York Times.*

The first time I stated that Canada's health care system was nothing more than an insurance scheme (and a badly run one at that) was during an appearance on Charles Adler's *Sun News* TV show in 2012 (youtube.com /watch?v=FviCxpy_9Oo).

There are too many books about nutrition, wellness, and prevention to list here. I'd suggest you simply visit your local bookstore or your favourite website for more information. One article on the subject ("Will we have a health care system or a sick care system? A tale of two futures") that I found helpful was written by John Auerbach and appeared in the March 21, 2013, edition of the *Huffington Post*.

Finding a family doctor and dealing with wait-lists. These two issues lie at the heart of what's wrong with Canada's health care system. The article that best sums up Canadians' frustrations with searching out a family practitioner to look after them and their families ("The soul-destroying search for a family doctor") was written by Gloria Galloway and appeared in the August 21, 2011, edition of the *Globe and Mail*. Global News and CTV News provided in-depth and unbiased coverage of the Fraser Institute's 2016 survey on wait times, which I refer to throughout this particular section of the book.

The introduction of a Canada-wide pharmacare program continues to evolve. Ontario's health minister, Dr. Eric Hoskins, resigned in the spring of 2018 and announced he wouldn't be running in the upcoming provincial election in order to chair a federal government advisory council with the goal of creating a new national pharmacare plan. As a result of this, I decided to concentrate more on eyes and teeth and less on the need to cover prescription drugs. Articles by Rosa Marchitelli ("Boy told he'd have to go blind before health system would pay for sight-saving surgery"), which was posted on the CBC News website on March 7, 2016, and Jacquie Maund and Hazel Stewart ("Why doesn't our health-care system cover dental?"), which appeared in the April 7, 2017, edition of the *Huffington Post*, and an editorial ("Canada doesn't have your back: Free health care only goes so far, especially for some seniors") that appeared in the September 8, 2014, edition of the *Financial Post* proved most invaluable.

Readers who wish to learn more about the internet's influence upon modern medicine are invited to pick up Dr. Eric Topol's book, *The Patient Will See You Now: The Future of Medicine is in Your Hands* (New York: Basic Books, 2015). Those wishing to check out Richard Worzel's many excellent books, including *The Next 20 Years of Your Life: A Personal Guide into the Year 2017* (Toronto: Stoddart, 1998) and *Who Owns Tomorrow? 7 Secrets for the Future of Business* (Toronto: Viking, 2003), as well as his blog, should visit his website at futuresearch.com. Richard is one of this country's brightest minds and I feel fortunate to count him among my friends.

The section entitled Cancer Inc. was based upon two articles I wrote that appeared in two different publications. The first ("War on cancer, like the one on drugs, has failed us") appeared in the July 11, 2016, edition of the *Hamilton Spectator*. The second ("It's time to end the Terry Fox Run and let the hero rest in peace") appeared in the November 29, 2013, edition of the *London Free Press*. To learn more about the Terry Fox Foundation, please visit terryfox.org.

The section entitled Medical Assistance in Dying was mostly comprised of an article I wrote ("Killing me softly") that appeared in the September 17, 2014, edition of the *Hamilton Spectator*. The various stories involving assisted suicide were culled from a bunch of sources, too numerous to mention. The author nonetheless expresses his gratitude to everyone involved with this issue, particularly Dr. Donald Low for the touching video he made on physician-assisted death just days before he died.

Those interested in reading the Kurt Vonnegut story referenced ("2 B R 0 2 B") can find it at gutenberg.org/ebooks/21279.

I first wrote about the three health care tsunamis in an article ("Boomers, zoomers and loomers: Impact of demographic shift on health-care will be massive") published in the April 9, 2016, edition of the *Hamilton Spectator*. The statistics cited come from a wide variety of sources, including the Canadian Obesity Network, the Canadian Diabetes Association, and the Alzheimer Society of Canada. To learn more about boomers and zoomers please visit everythingzoomer.com.

An Interlude: The Hypocritical Oath

The Hippocratic oath is a pledge that physicians take upon finishing their medical education before becoming doctors. Although the ancient text is only of historic and symbolic value, swearing the oath remains a rite of passage for medical graduates around the world. As a result, Hippocrates is often referred to as the "father of medicine" in many countries.

I initially explored the topic of doctors and the Stockholm Syndrome when I published an article in the May 31, 2013, edition of the *Kingston Whig-Standard* ("A revolution brewing among Ontario's doctors"). In researching the phenomenon of Stockholm Syndrome, I found an article by Kathryn Westcott, "What is Stockholm syndrome?," *BBC News Magazine*, August 22, 2013, to be most enlightening.

An earlier version of the story detailing how Dr. Anthony Hsu was audited to death appeared in the April 5, 2012, edition of the *Medical Post* ("The real heroes behind the dismantling of Ontario's MRC") under my name. Christie Blatchford wrote a number of superb articles for the *Globe and Mail* in the autumn of 2004 ("The farce and tragedy of medical audits" and "Gentle Dr. Hsu and the audit that haunted him") and spring of 2005 ("Audit system 'devastating' for MDs") that helped shine a light on the nefarious doings of the CPSO's Medical Review Committee. Dr. Barry Dworkin also wrote a poignant piece ("Death of caring doctor should concern all Canadians") that appeared in the April 22, 2003, edition of the *Ottawa Citizen* shortly after Dr. Hsu's body was discovered.

The Reign of Terror refers to a period during the French Revolution when suspected enemies of the Revolution were captured and brutally executed.

An insightful article on Dr. Eric Hoskins's negative influence on Ontario's health care system ("Health care has crumbled under Eric Hoskins' watch") was written by Dr. Sohail Gandhi and appeared in the April 24, 2017, edition of the *Huffington Post*. Another great piece detailing the battle between Ontario's doctors and health minister Hoskins ("Better pay for doctors won't cure what ails the system") appeared in the June 26, 2017, edition of the *Toronto Star* under Martin Regg Cohn's byline. Carly Weeks also chimed in on the issue, penning an article ("Ontario must clamp down on high-billing doctors, health minister says") in the April 22, 2016, edition of the *Globe and Mail*.

To learn more about Health Minister Jane Philpott's appearance at the 150th annual meeting of the Canadian Medical Association, readers may wish to take a look at André Picard's column ("Health Minister Jane Philpott urges physicians to use power, privilege to help Canada's vulnerable") in the August 21, 2017, edition of the *Globe and Mail*.

Conversion on the road to Damascus refers to the conversion of Saul/Paul to Christianity while travelling to Damascus. In modern times, it most often references a turning point in someone's life, in which a reversal of some pre-existing beliefs or ideas occurs.

Dr. Charles Shaver wrote a tremendous article ("Morneau's tax plan poses risk for doctors and dentists") in the October 16, 2017, edition of the *Ottawa Citizen* examining the negative effects federal finance minister Bill Morneau's proposed changes to the tax system would have on both doctors and dentists.

Part III: First, Do No Harm

The promise to "first, do no harm" (in the Latin version, "*primum non nocere*") supposedly was uttered by Hippocrates many centuries ago.

As part of my research, I read a number of especially instructive articles about midwives and nurse practitioners. One of the best was written by Michele Sponagle ("The Nurse Practitioner Will See You Now") and appeared in the March 2011 edition of *Canadian Living* magazine. A second article ("Midwives: Underused and misused assets in Canada") was written by André Picard and first appeared in the July 10, 2013, edition of the *Globe and Mail*. Another article ("Nurse practitioners in Canada more than double in five years") that proved particularly useful in helping me understand the role of nurse practitioners was also written by André Picard and appeared in the January 26, 2012, edition of the *Globe and Mail*.

For the section on primary care reform, I drew heavily upon my own experiences lobbying the issue for the Ontario Medical Association in the late 1990s. However, there are a number of articles that I also found enlightening. These include a piece ("Ontario's curious shift away from family health teams") written by Kelly Grant that appeared in the February 15, 2015, edition of the *Globe and Mail* and another ("Ontario's bold bet on health-care reform") penned by Bob Hepburn that graced the pages of the June 5, 2016, *Toronto Star*. Readers may also wish to visit the healthydebate.ca website, where a piece co-authored by Vanessa Milne, Michael Nolan, and Jeremy Petch ("The Price-Baker report: What does it mean for primary care reform in Ontario?") was posted on November 19, 2015.

I'd also be remiss if I didn't thank Dr. Wendy Graham, primary care reform's leading proponent, who spent many hours over the years patiently going over the ins and outs of primary care reform with me, as well as explaining why it's necessary the government reforms how we deliver primary care if we're to have any hope of saving family practice in Ontario and elsewhere in Canada.

The American writer Joseph Heller had a line in one of his books, *Good as Gold* (New York: Simon & Schuster, 1979), that went something like this: "Nothing succeeds like failure and nothing fails like success." Having spent the past two decades as a witness to the EMR follies, I can't help wondering if Heller wasn't thinking about the province of Ontario and its experience with electronic medical records. In recounting this sad, shameful saga, I leaned on a number of articles, including: "Why eHealth went 'off the rails'" by Tanya Talaga, which appeared in the October 10, 2009, edition of the *Toronto Star*, and a Canadian Press story ("Ontario Tories say eHealth still wasting billions of dollars, three years after scathing auditor-general report") that appeared in the July 23, 2012, edition of the *National Post*. Two other articles, "The real eHealth Ontario scandal isn't over Choco Bites" (written by André Picard for the *Globe and Mail* on June 24, 2009) and "Report: Ontario patients should have access to electronic medical records" (written by Keith Leslie for the Canadian Press on November 22, 2016), were also helpful.

I've written numerous articles about the Ontario Liberals and their disastrous Transformation Agenda. A piece ("Health care on its death bed") that appeared in the July 3, 2015, edition of the *London Free Press* pretty much says it all. For a doctor's perspective on Dr. Eric Hoskins and his efforts to drive the last stake through the heart of health care in Ontario, I'd suggest readers check out an article ("Desperation is setting in for the Ontario Liberals") written by Dr. Sohail Gandhi, which appeared in the March 28, 2016, edition of the *Huffington Post*. Last but not least, an interview with health minister George Smitherman conducted by Ken Tremblay ("Insight: In conversation with George Smitherman") that appeared in the September 2006 edition of *Healthcare Quarterly* is nothing if not enlightening on the topic of transforming the province's health care system.

An especially insightful article on the Choosing Wisely initiative ("Is Canada health care choosing wisely?") was written by Dr. Adam Kassam and can be found in the October 16, 2017, edition of the *Toronto Star*. To further supplement your understanding of the issue, I'd recommend you read the following two articles: "Unnecessary care in Canada tops 1 million tests and treatments a year" by Amina Zafar, which was posted to the CBC News website on April 6, 2017, and "Medical groups produce list of overused tests in 'Choosing Wisely' campaign," which was authored by Helen Branswell of the Canadian Press and appeared on April 3, 2014.

Those wishing to learn more about choosing wisely may wish to explore their website at choosingwiselycanada.org.

Part IV: The Big Fix

The Big Fix is the name of a 1947 American crime thriller directed by James Flood. In 1978, another film, this time a comedy-thriller directed by Jeremy Kagan, also appeared under this name. Finally, a 2012 documentary dealing with the Deepwater Horizon oil spill was released, also bearing the name *The Big Fix*.

Many of the ideas in Part IV: "The Big Fix" were initially discussed in a series of articles I wrote between 2012 and 2016. First up was an article ("Five myths about health care") that appeared in the July 29, 2012, edition of the *Kingston Whig-Standard*. Next came one ("Canada's health-care system is ailing and needs to be resuscitated before it's too late") that appeared in the December 5, 2014, edition of the *London Free Press*. This was followed by "Cure for what ails it," which appeared in the March 20, 2015, edition of the same paper. The *Hamilton Spectator* then published "Dear Premier Wynne: Health care is a bloody mess" on January 15, 2015. A year and a half later, another piece written by me ("Imaginative, honest talk is missing as politicians tackle a new Health Care Accord") was published in the August 26, 2016, edition of the *London Free Press*. Shortly thereafter, a follow-up column ("The Big Fix") appeared in the October 20, 2016, edition of the *Timmins Press*.

The best definition of evidence-based medicine I've found comes from Dr. David Sackett, a Canadian doctor considered to be one of the fathers of evidence-based medicine, who says it's "the conscientious, explicit and judicious use of current best evidence in making decisions about the care of the individual patient."

Just about every Canadian knows the Canada Health Act consists of five main principles: (1) public administration, (2) comprehensiveness, (3) universality, (4) portability, and (5) accessibility. But did you know that, in addition to these five, Tommy Douglas's version of medicare had three more: (1) effective, (2) efficient, and (3) responsible? Sadly, Justice Emmett Hall decided not to include these last three principles when he made his recommendations to the federal government in the early 1960s. It's also worth noting that Tommy Douglas never intended for the government to solely control the delivery of health care.

Although there's no clear consensus regarding the origin of the phrase "If you don't stand for something, you'll fall for anything," most attribute it to Alexander Hamilton.

For those interested in learning more about former Ontario premiers John Robarts and Bill Davis, I'd direct your attention to two fine books by Steve Paikin: *Public Triumph, Private Tragedy: The Double Life of John P. Robarts* (Toronto: Viking, 2005) and *Bill Davis: Nation Builder, and Not So Bland After All* (Toronto: Dundurn, 2016). To further supplement your knowledge of the Ontario political scene post-1985, readers are encouraged to take a look at two other seminal books: *Ontario Since 1985* by Randall White (Toronto: Venture Press, 1998) and *Cycling into Saigon: The Conservative Transition in Ontario* by David R. Cameron and Graham White (Vancouver: UBC Press, 2000).

There are a number of articles about the Patients First Act, including one by Dr. Nadia Alam ("Ontario Doctors Like Me Won't Play Along with Patients First Act") that appeared in the September 12, 2016, edition of the *Huffington Post* and another by Dr. Sohail Gandhi ("Ontario's Patients First Act is a Flashback to the Disastrous '90s") that ran in the September 25, 2016, edition of the same publication. Similarly, a thoughtful piece detailing the problems with the Protecting Patients Act written by Lonny Rosen and Elyse Sunshine ("New patient protection law must allow sentencing discretion") appeared in the January 11, 2017, edition of the *Toronto Star*.

Those interested in learning more about patient-centred care should visit the website of an organization led by Dr. Vaughan Glover known as the Canadian Association for Person-Centred Health at capch.org.

To learn more about Health Quality Ontario, or to download the document *Quality Matters: Realizing Excellent Care for All*, please visit their website at hqontario.ca.

A number of articles appeared following the death of Ontario teenager Laura Hillier. The one I leaned on the most was written by Diana Zlomislic ("Plea from dying teen: Please help"), which appeared in the April 23, 2016, edition of the *Toronto Star*. In telling the tragic tale of young Walid Khalfallah, I relied upon the reporting of Pamela Fayerman, whose article ("Mother of boy paralyzed after surgery delays throws support behind private clinic owner's lawsuit") appeared in the November 15, 2012, edition of the *Vancouver Sun*. Lisa Johnson wrote an outstanding article detailing the plight of little Meghan Arnott ("'Kids are in pain' waiting for postponed surgeries at B.C. Children's Hospital, mom says"), which was first posted to the CBC News website on May 10, 2016.

An obituary written by Stephanie Hernandez McGavin ("Robert Cox, ad man behind Ford's 'Quality is Job 1' pitch, dies") that appeared in the June 29, 2016, edition of the *Automotive News* was of great use in my getting the facts straight about the origin of Ford's advertising campaign.

As if having fourteen health ministries in Canada wasn't already bad enough, Prime Minister Trudeau named former health minister Jane Philpott the new minister of Indigenous Services on August 28, 2017. The new ministry will primarily be responsible for ensuring First Nations Canadians have a say in the kinds of health care services and treatments they receive.

For a breakdown of the separation of powers and responsibilities between the federal government and provincial and territorial governments, I'd recommend readers check out canada.ca/en/intergovernmental-affairs.

An article by Dr. Jean Marmoreo ("We're still not as fit as Swedes, but we shouldn't stop trying") that appeared in the January 28, 2015, edition of the *Globe and Mail* was especially helpful to me in bringing the saga of the sixty-year-old Swede and the thirty-year-old Canadian up to date. Another article by Laurie Monsebraaten ("Prescription for healthier population: Spend more on social services") that was published in the *Toronto Star* on January 22, 2018, provided invaluable details regarding a study by Dr. Daniel Dutton of the School of Public Policy at the University of Calgary on the effect that spending on social programs has on keeping health care costs down.

Those looking to learn more about alternative cancer therapies in Canada would be well advised to contact Dr. Akbar Khan, who can be reached at medicorcancer.com.

An article on the CTV News website ("63,000 Canadians left the country for medical treatment last year: Fraser Institute"), posted on July 2, 2017, was instrumental in allowing me to develop my ideas with regards to medical tourism. A second article written by Dan Fumano ("The dark side of medical tourism: How quick and cheap treatment abroad can prove costly to health, and our health-care system") that ran in the April 25, 2016, edition of the *Vancouver Sun* helped me better understand the political battle over medical tourism that continues to rage in British Columbia and, indeed, the rest of our country.

The line about "never missing an opportunity to miss an opportunity" originally came from Abba Eban, an Israeli diplomat, politician, and author, following the Geneva Peace Conference in 1973.

The *Hamilton Spectator* published a great series of stories in the winter of 2017 as part of an investigative report into the problem of "bed-blockers" clogging up hospital emergency departments in the province of Ontario that I enjoyed immensely. Another article ("Ontario's Patient Ombudsman eyes improvements to health care") written by Shawn Jeffords of the Canadian Press on November 9, 2017, also shone light on the overcrowding problem.

I first learned about medical savings accounts while reading Dr. David Gratzer's fine book *Code Blue: Reviving Canada's Health Care System* (Toronto: ECW Press, 1999).

An earlier version of my interview with Dr. Brian Day ("Tommy Douglas 'would not be happy' with our system: Dr. Brian Day on his fight for medicare freedom") appeared in the September 8, 2016, edition of the *Financial Post*. To learn more about Dr. Day, please visit his website at brianday.ca. Those interested in making a donation to help fund Dr. Day's Charter challenge in British Columbia are urged to go to ccf.formstack.com/forms/health_cant_wait_donation.

To discover why the defenders of the status quo are so afraid of Dr. Day and Dr. Chaoulli, I'd recommend reading an article ("The dangerous ideas of Dr. Jacques Chaoulli") by Margaret Wente that appeared in the June 8, 2004, edition of the *Globe and Mail*.

To the best of my memory, the first person who uttered the phrase "Fund it or free it" within my earshot was former Ontario Medical Association president Dr. Kenneth Sky. Dr. Sky, one of Toronto's top ear, nose, and throat doctors, was a fierce advocate for the hybrid solution and possessed a wicked sense of humour, often referring to himself as "an ear, nose, and *wallet* doctor," which needless to say drove politically correct OMA staffers crazy.

Coda: "That's All, Folks!"

"That's all, folks!" made its first appearance at the conclusion of a 1930 Warner Brothers *Looney Tunes* cartoon and was spoken by a character named Bosko. While a number of other characters have delivered the line over the years, the most famous to do so was undoubtedly Porky Pig. "That's all, folks!" is so popular it even adorns Mel Blanc's grave marker. Blanc was the voice of Porky Pig, along with many other characters.

I first wrote about the need for a health care revolution here in Canada when I published an article in the February 14, 2017, edition of the *Ottawa Citizen* ("Canada needs an 'Arab Spring' in health care"). In the article, I suggested that the citizens of Canada need to rise up and take back our health care system before our elected officials and civil servants can do any more damage. For those who don't remember, the term "Arab Spring" refers to an outbreak of both violent and non-violent demonstrations in North Africa and the Middle East that began on December 18, 2010, in Tunisia. As for the origin of the term itself, "Arab Spring" is thought to be an allusion to the revolutions of 1848, which are collectively referred to as the "Springtime of Nations," as well as 1968's Prague Spring.

Although Albert Einstein is generally credited with coming up with the line "Insanity is doing the same thing over and over again and expecting different results," there's no clear evidence that it originated with him or that he even uttered those words at any time in his life.

The cha-cha-cha is a dance of Cuban origin that was introduced in the early 1950s by composer and violinist Enrique Jorrin. The name of the dance is derived from the shuffling sound of the dancers' feet.

Freedom 55 is the name of a program introduced by London Life Insurance Company back in the late 1980s. The idea was that by following their prudent financial advice, you'd be able to retire early, ideally at age fifty-five.

INDEX

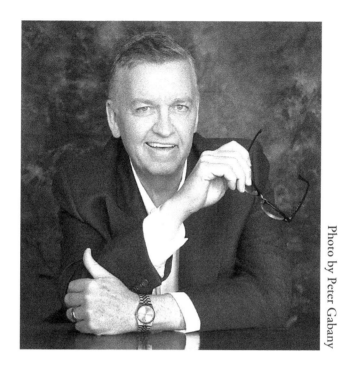

Photo by Peter Gabany

ABOUT THE AUTHOR

Stephen Skyvington is one of Canada's pre-eminent political pundits and health care policy experts. His columns regularly appear in newspapers all across Canada, under the banner Opinions and Observations. Stephen also appears on NEWSTALK 1010 with Ted Woloshyn every Saturday afternoon. Formerly the manager of government relations for the Ontario Medical Association, where he spent six and a half years lobbying elected officials and civil servants at all three levels of government, Stephen is currently the president of PoliTrain Inc., a public relations firm he founded in 2001, specializing in leadership development and candidate training, lobbying, and crisis management. In addition to being a full-time registered lobbyist, Stephen, who has been involved in politics since 1988, also has a great deal of experience in community and stakeholder relations, as well as media and government relations. He lives in Cobourg, Ontario.

Book Credits
Developmental Editor: Dominic Farrell
Project Editor: Jenny McWha
Copy Editor: Laurie Miller
Proofreader: Ashley Hisson
Indexer: Sergey Lobachev

Cover Designer: Laura Boyle
Interior Designer: Sophie Paas-Lang

Publicist: Tabassum Siddiqui

Dundurn
Publisher: J. Kirk Howard
Vice-President: Carl A. Brand
Editorial Director: Kathryn Lane
Artistic Director: Laura Boyle
Production Manager: Rudi Garcia
Publicity Manager: Michelle Melski
Manager, Accounting and Technical Services: Livio Copetti

Editorial: Allison Hirst, Dominic Farrell, Jenny McWha, Rachel Spence,
Elena Radic, Melissa Kawaguchi
Marketing and Publicity: Kendra Martin, Elham Ali,
Tabassum Siddiqui, Heather McLeod
Design and Production: Sophie Paas-Lang

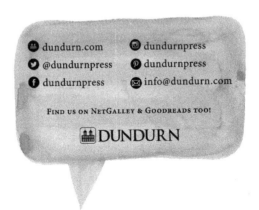

dundurn.com dundurnpress
@dundurnpress dundurnpress
dundurnpress info@dundurn.com

FIND US ON NETGALLEY & GOODREADS TOO!

DUNDURN